Essentials in Ophthalmology

Uveitis and Immunological Disorders

U. Pleyer   J.V. Forrester

Editors

Essentials in Ophthalmology

G. K. Krieglstein   R. N. Weinreb
Series Editors

Glaucoma

Cataract and Refractive Surgery

Uveitis and Immunological Disorders

Vitreo-retinal Surgery

Medical Retina

Oculoplastics and Orbit

**Pediatric Ophthalmology,
Neuro-Ophthalmology, Genetics**

Cornea and External Eye Disease

Editors Uwe Pleyer
John V. Forrester

Uveitis and Immunological Disorders

Progress III

With 30 Figures, Mostly in Colour
and 9 Tables

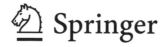 Springer

Series Editors

Günter K. Krieglstein, MD
Professor and Chairman
Department of Ophthalmology
University of Cologne
Kerpener Straße 62
50924 Cologne
Germany

Robert N. Weinreb, MD
Professor and Director
Hamilton Glaucoma Center
Department of Ophthalmology
University of California at San Diego
9500 Gilman Drive
La Jolla, CA 92093-0946
USA

Volume Editors

Uwe Pleyer, MD
Professor of Ophthalmology
Universitätsklinikum Berlin
Charité
Department of Ophthalmology
Augustenburger Straße 1
13353 Berlin
Germany

John V. Forrester, MD, FRCSE, FRCSG, FRC Ophth
Cockburn Professor and Head of Department
Department of Ophthalmology
Institute of Medical Sciences, Foresterhill
University of Aberdeen
Aberdeen, AB25 2ZD
Scotland
UK

ISBN 978-3-540-69458-8   e-ISBN 978-3-540-69459-5

ISSN 1612-3212

Library of Congress Control Number: 2008932108

Cover Design: WMXDesign GmbH, Heidelberg, Germany

Printed on acid-free paper

9 8 7 6 5 4 3 2 1

springer.com

Foreword

The Essentials in Ophthalmology series represents an unique updating publication on the progress in all subspecialties of ophthalmology.

In a quarterly rhythm, eight issues are published covering clinically relevant achievements in the whole field of ophthalmology. This timely transfer of advancements for the best possible care of our eye patients has proven to be effective. The initial working hypothesis of providing new knowledge immediately following publication in the peer-reviewed journal and not waiting for the textbook appears to be highly workable.

We are now entering the third cycle of the Essentials in Ophthalmology series, having been encouraged by readership acceptance of the first two series, each of eight volumes. This is a success that was made possible predominantly by the numerous opinion-leading authors and the outstanding section editors, as well as with the constructive support of the publisher. There are many good reasons to continue andstill improve the dissemination of this didactic and clinically relevant information.

G.K. Krieglstein
R.N. Weinreb
Series Editors

Preface

Our knowledge and understanding of immune-mediated diseases has increased exponentially over the past few years, especially in the areas of immunopathogenesis and immunotherapeutics. Uveitis is one of the most common potentially blinding disorders, and one that is often underestimated but is now considered a leading cause of severe eye damage, particularly in younger age groups. Over the past few years, immune-mediated mechanisms—both innate and adaptive—have also been implicated in other disorders, such as diabetic retinopathy and macular degeneration.

This third volume of Uveitis and Immunological Disorders in the Essentials in Ophthalmology series provides the ophthalmologist with practical information on current diagnostic and therapeutic aspects of several ocular disorders from the front to the back of the eye. In addition, there are important discussions of the mechanisms underlying these conditions, which incorporate the most recent research material available. The scope of the chapters ranges from well-recognized immune disorders such as cornea transplantation, uveitis and diabetic retinopathy, to less well recognized but newly emerging immunologically linked diseases, such as macular degeneration. This book covers, in particular, new aspects of HLA-B27-associated anterior uveitis, keratouveitis, and steroid sensitivity in uveitis patients. Further emphasis is placed on the nature of the intraocular inflammation and systemic disorders such as Behçet's vasculitis and multiple sclerosis.

We are grateful to all of the authors that have contributed to this edition of Uveitis and Immunological Disorders. We are sure that this book will find its audience, and we hope that it will serve in the interest of many patients.

Uwe Pleyer
John V. Forrester

Contents

Contributors

Daniel Böhringer
University of Freiburg
Department of Opthalmology
Killianstraße 5
79106 Freiburg, Germany

John H. Chang
Laboratory of Ocular Immunology
Inflammatory Diseases Research Unit
School of Medical Sciences
University of New South Wales
Sydney, Australia
and
Department of Ophthalmology
St Vincent's Hospital
Sydney, Australia

S. John Curnow
Institute of Biomedical Research
Division of Immunity and Infection
Medical School
The University of Birmingham
Birmingham B15 2TT, UK

A.K.O. Denniston
Institute of Biomedical Research
MRC Centre for Immune Regulation
Division of Immunity and Infection
Medical School, The University of Birmingham
Birmingham B15 2TT, UK;
Academic Unit of Ophthalmology
Division of Immunity and Infection
Birmingham and Midland Eye Centre
University of Birmingham
City Hospital NHS Trust
Birmingham B18 7QU, UK

Andrew D. Dick
Academic Unit of Ophthalmology
University of Bristol and Bristol Eye Hospital
Lower Maudlin Street
Bristol BS1 2LX, UK

John V. Forrester
Department of Ophthalmology
Institute of Medical Sciences, Foresterhill
University of Aberdeen
Aberdeen, AB 25 2ZD
Scotland, UK

F. Goezinne
Eye Research Institute Maastricht
Department of Ophthalmology
University Hospital Maastricht
P. Debyelaan 25, 6202 AZ, Maastricht
The Netherlands

Elizabeth Graham
Department of Ophthalmology
Guy's & St. Thomas' NHS Trust
London, UK

F. Hendrikse
Eye Research Institute Maastricht
Department of Ophthalmology
University Hospital Maastricht
P. Debyelaan 25, 6202 AZ, Maastricht
The Netherlands

Antonia M. Joussen
Department of Ophthalmology
University of Duesseldorf
Moorenstrabe 5, 40225 Duesseldorf
Germany

A. Kijlstra
Eye Research Institute Maastricht
Department of Ophthalmology
University Hospital Maastricht
P. Debyelaan 25, 6202 AZ, Maastricht
The Netherlands

E.C. La Heij
Eye Research Institute Maastricht
Department of Ophthalmology
University Hospital Maastricht
P. Debyelaan 25, 6202 AZ, Maastricht
The Netherlands

Richard W.J. Lee
Academic Unit of Ophthalmology
University of Bristol and Bristol Eye Hospital
Lower Maudlin Street
Bristol BS1 2LX, UK

Rashmi Mathew
Department of Ophthalmology
Medical Eye Unit
St Thomas' Hospital
London SE1 7EH, UK

Peter J. McCluskey
Laboratory of Ocular Immunology
Inflammatory Diseases Research Unit
School of Medical Sciences
University of New South Wales
Sydney, Australia
and
Department of Ophthalmology
St Vincent's Hospital
Sydney, Australia
and
Department of Ophthalmology
Royal Prince Alfred Hospital
Sydney, Australia

Ben J.E. Raveney
Academic Unit of Ophthalmology
University of Bristol and Bristol Eye Hospital
Lower Maudlin Street
Bristol BS1 2LX, UK

T. Reinhard
University of Freiburg
Department of Opthalmology
Killianstraße 5
79106 Freiburg, Germany

Shouvik Saha
Department of Ophthalmology
Guy's & St. Thomas' NHS Trust
London, UK

Lauren P. Schewitz
Academic Unit of Ophthalmology
University of Bristol and Bristol Eye Hospital
Lower Maudlin Street
Bristol BS1 2LX, UK

Miles Stanford
St Thomas' Hospital
Department of Clinical Ophthalmology
Medical Eye Unit
London SE1 7EH, UK

Denis Wakefield
Laboratory of Ocular Immunology
Inflammatory Diseases Research Unit
School of Medical Sciences
University of New South Wales
Sydney, Australia and
Department of Ophthalmology
St Vincent's Hospital
Sydney, Australia

Graeme J. Williams
Diabetes Retinal Screening Service
David Anderson Building
Foresterhill Road
Aberdeen, AB25 2ZP
UK

Heping Xu
Department of Ophthalmology
Inflammation and Immunity Theme
School of Medicine
Institute of Medical Sciences (IMS)
University of Aberdeen, Foresterhill
Aberdeen, AB25 2ZD
Scotland, UK

Chapter 1

Histocompatibility Matching in Penetrating Keratoplasty

1

Daniel Böhringer, Thomas Reinhard

Core Messages

- HLA matching reduces graft rejections in normal-risk as well as in high-risk keratoplasty.
- Most patients can be served with an HLA-compatible graft within well under a year, even if they are on a monocenter waiting list.
- Waiting times for a histocompatible graft can be predicted and discussed with each patient in advance.
- The HLAMatchmaker algorithm can balance waiting time and histocompatibility for patients with poor match ability.

- The HLA-A1/H-Y minor antigen causes immunogenicity comparable to HLA mismatches: allocating male HLA-A1-positive donors to female recipients should be avoided.
- Matching of ABO blood group antigens is warranted in high-risk keratoplasty.
- Long-term graft survival will most likely improve upon the routine matching of major and selected minor histocompatibility antigens. This strategy will outweigh the cost of HLA typing in the long run.

1.1 Introduction

In this chapter, recent developments in histocompatibility matching for penetrating keratoplasty are presented and a strategy for clinical practice is recommended.

Despite the immune privilege in the anterior chamber of the eye, graft rejections are a major complication of penetrating keratoplasty, as they facilitate subsequent graft failure. The application of topical corticosteroids for several months has commonly been thought to be sufficiently protective. Nevertheless, on average, 18% of normal-risk keratoplasty cases [18] and up to 75% of high-risk cases [20] experience immune reactions. The life expectancy of affected grafts is significantly reduced due to immunologic endothelial cell loss. In normal risk cases, immune reactions accumulate in the first two years. However, most high-risk cases are at persistent risk of graft reactions. This risk can be reduced by means of intensified and prolonged prophylaxis with topical corticosteroids and with systemic immunosuppression [19]. The protective effect, however, ceases upon discontinuation of the immunosuppressive regimen. Any long-term dependence on immunosuppression is associated with additional costs and potentially serious side effects. Donor selection by avoiding graft antigens foreign to the recipient is termed "antigen matching" or "histocompatibility." Matching of human leukocyte antigens (HLA matching, Sect. 1.2) and more recently another antigen system (minor matching, Sect. 1.3) both have the potential to primarily and permanently avoiding immune reactions, as is the case in autologous keratoplasty.

Summary for the Clinician

- Unlike immunosuppression, histocompatibility can permanently reduce graft rejections

1.2 Major Transplantation Antigens (HLA)

The experimental transfer of tumours from one mouse strain to others led to the discovery of the major histocompatibility complex (MHC). In humans, these antigens were discovered after a multiparous woman suffered a transfusion reaction despite blood group compatibility. The human MHC equivalent was subsequently termed human leukocyte antigen (HLA). This highly polymorphic antigen system comprises of more than ten gene loci on chromosome 6. Theoretically, more than one million different individual combinations of the known alleles at the HLA loci A, B and DR could exist. However, only a small fraction are actually observed due to strong linkage disequilibrium. This subset of phenotypes comprises population-specific haplotypes.

The gene loci from the HLA systems are functionally subdivided into two classes according to the pattern of their expression on the cellular surface:

- Class I molecules are expressed on almost all nucleated cells. They comprise a heavy chain, a light chain (beta-2 microglobulin) and a small peptide of nine amino-acid residues. This peptide is termed a "minor antigen" (Sect. 1.3), and is derived from degraded cytosolic proteins. Three gene loci of major importance have been identified for class I: HLA-A, HLA-B and HLA-C. Further loci are termed C, E, F, G, K and L. These additional loci are deemed less important for transplantation medicine, as they are either strongly genetically linked to the A/B haplotypes or not associated with high allelic polymorphism.
- Class II molecules are homodimers. These molecules are exclusively expressed on cells that share the ability to present extracellular antigens to the immune system (e.g., monocyte- and lymphocyte-derived strains). The HLA class II locus of major immunologic importance is HLA-DR. Further loci that are deemed of less independent importance are HLA-DP, DQ, DM and DO.

1.2.1 Typing Methods

HLA antigens were discovered by means of serological assays. Only the macro agglutination assay was available initially. For this assay, patient serum was mixed with test cells bearing only the respective antigen. Any macroscopically visible agglutination demonstrated the presence of antibodies directed against the respective test cells. Depending on the availability of appropriate test cells, only a subset of all HLA antibodies could be detected at that time. Current serologic methods of HLA typing are based on the complement-dependent cytotoxicity assay (CDC). For HLA typing, cells are incubated against a battery of standardized antibodies as defined by the International Histocompatibility Workshop (IHW).

The first generation of CDC test sera were unable to detect differences of only a few amino acid residues between certain HLA alleles. When monoclonal antibody techniques became available, the IHW released a new generation of test sera that were eventually able to split most of the alleles known at that time into specific subgroups. As the HLA nomenclature was already established at that time, the newly discovered alleles were termed "splits" of the established "broad" antigens and were sequentially assigned running allele numbers.

Further improvements in HLA typing were achieved by means of molecular techniques: the polymerase chain reaction (PCR) can specifically detect small parts of the genome by means of specific primers and subsequent amplification reactions. HLA typing is achieved either by sequence-specific oligonucleotide priming, where alleles are identified by characteristic "fingerprint" sequences, or by sequence typing of the whole allele (which is more expensive). These approaches led to the discovery of more than 100 HLA alleles on each of the HLA loci A, B and DR. For example, the broad antigen HLA DR3 can be divided into the split antigens DR17 and DR18, which in turn can be subdivided into DRB1*0302 and DRB1*0303 at the molecular level.

In corneal transplantation, blood for HLA typing is commonly collected after the donor's death. Due to autolytic changes, the amount of viable cells available for serologic analysis is often insufficient. In this situation, molecular methods can still detect the HLA phenotype with excellent precision, whereas serologic techniques depend on viable cells and are not likely to detect all donor antigens.

Summary for the Clinician

- Various HLA molecules are omnipresent on the cellular surface
- More than 100 alleles have been identified at each HLA locus
- Only a small fraction of all possible permutations of the alleles at the HLA loci A, B and DR are actually observable and comprise population-specific haplotypes
- HLA typing should be performed using molecular techniques due to their high accuracy and optimal allele resolution

---

1.2.2 Discussion of the Evidence for HLA Matching in Penetrating Keratoplasty

The potential of HLA matching for prophylaxis of immune reactions is currently largely unexploited in penetrating keratoplasty, as the clinical evidence is contradictory at first sight: the only randomized clinical trial (CCTS) failed to demonstrate a significant protective effect of HLA matching in penetrating keratoplasty [23]. By contrast, most recent investigations on large homogeneous cohorts report substantial protection from HLA compatibility [2, 16, 18, 20, 24]. Two major explanations for this contradiction have been identified:

1. The major problem with the CCTS was inaccurate HLA typing. The analysis was based on typing data

that differed from retyping with molecular techniques in 55% [13]. The importance of highly accurate HLA typing for successful HLA matching was systematically investigated by means of statistical simulation analysis: even 5% faulty HLA DR typing made a beneficial matching effect undetectable [24].

2. High dosages of topical immunosuppression from the CCTS protocol for postoperative medical aftercare rendered the detection of any HLA effect unlikely.

Both issues were overcome in more recent investigations on HLA matching in penetrating keratoplasty. These studies uniformly demonstrate a beneficial effect of HLA matching with respect to immune reactions. Additional lessons about the efficacy of HLA matching can be learned from three of them:

- In 1,681 consecutive transplantations from just one center, there was a benefit from additionally matching the class II locus HLA-DR to the class I loci A and B [24]
- A beneficial effect from class I matching alone is only observed when matching is based on split rather than broad (see Sect. 1.2.1) HLA alleles [2] in high-risk cases
- HLA matching of HLA A, B and DR broad alleles is beneficial in normal-risk keratoplasty (first keratoplasty for bullous keratopathy, Fuchs' endothelial dystrophy, keratoconus with centrally sutured graft or avascular corneal scars): after four years, the group with up to two mismatches experienced 25% fewer immune reactions than those bearing 3–6 mismatches [18]

Summary for the Clinician

- A mounting body of evidence supports the beneficial effects of HLA matching in normal-risk as well as in high-risk keratoplasty
- The accuracy and precision of HLA typing is crucial to HLA matching

1.2.3   Differential HLA Matching

HLA mismatches differ in immunogenicity strength and thus in graft survival deterioration. This has long been observed in kidney transplantation [8] and in keratoplasty [7]. The structural basis of this phenomenon is well established for HLA class I loci [9]. This paved the way to the prediction of "acceptable" mismatches on an individual basis: the HLAMatchmaker algorithm defines nearly fifty omnipresent epitopes within the molecular structure of all HLA class I alleles. These epitopes are thought to be particularly exposed to the immune system and partitioned into triplets of amino-acid residues to account for the thermodynamic characteristics of the

antibody recognition reaction. All exposed amino-acid triplets are sequentially concatenated to form the triplet string for a particular allele. As the triplet string is derived from the primary structure of the HLA allele, it can be exclusively derived from molecular HLA typing.

The quality of matching is assessed by counting all triplets of the donor's triplet strings that are not identical to any of the corresponding triplets of the recipient's four triplet strings (two each for HLA-A and -B). HLA mismatches with zero to a few mismatched triplets are supposed to be fully histocompatible with regard to the antibody epitopes. Accordingly, it is known that they do not deteriorate graft survival in kidney transplantation [11]. A beneficial effect of this algorithm was also demonstrated recently in penetrating keratoplasty [4].

More recently, a first step towards HLA class II epitope matching has been made [10]. However, it is yet to be applied to penetrating keratoplasty.

Summary for the Clinician

- The HLAMatchmaker algorithm can help to identify HLA mismatches that are deemed mostly "harmless" with respect to immune reactions.
- HLAMatchmaker can help to provide histocompatible grafts to patients with rare HLA phenotypes within a reasonable time. Alternatively, the decreased waiting time could be traded for better match quality.

1.3   Minor (H) Transplantation Antigens

Graft rejections are even observed in HLA-identical allogeneic transplantations. These effects are ascribed to disparities in minor histocompatibility (H) antigens. In animal models, specific recognition of "foreign" H antigens by the host immune system has been demonstrated to elicit immune reactions [12]. A single H antigen mismatch even exceeds the immunogenicity of a single MHC mismatch in a mouse model for high-risk keratoplasty [25]. H antigens are peptides derived from polymorphic proteins of degraded cytosolic proteins. Their immunogenicity arises as a result of their presentation on the plasma membrane in the context of HLA class I or II, where they are recognized by alloreactive HLA-restricted T cells. The subset of cytosolic peptides that can bind to the HLA molecules strongly depends on the HLA allele (HLA restriction). In animal models, antigen-presenting cells (APC) such as limbal Langerhans cells have been demonstrated to migrate from the graft to the host spleen via the camero-splenic axis [17].

1

The spleen might thus be a source of a cytotoxic specific immune response directed against foreign graft H antigens presented by graft APCs. Recipient APCs might be an additional source of allogeneic minor antigens upon processing cellular graft detritus. Table 1.1 summarizes the H antigens that have recently been identified as being relevant to hematological transplantations [22]. However, only two of them (H-Y and HA-3) have been investigated in the context of corneal transplantation.

1.3.1 Discussion of Selected H Antigens

1.3.1.1 H-Y

Male grafts can be subject to alloimmune reactivity in female recipients, as antigens of the H-Y group are only expressed in male individuals and not in females. H-Y antigens are believed to occur in all tissues, including the human cornea. Epitopes of the H-Y antigen family are expressed in the context of either HLA-A1 or HLA-A2. The HLA-A1/H-Y antigen is located in the Y-chromosome-encoded DFFRY protein. The HLA-A*0201-restricted HLA-A2/H-Y antigen contains a post-translationally modified cysteine that significantly affects T cell recognition. A 20% reduction in graft rejections was recently demonstrated for 252 keratoplasties after matching the HLA-A1/H-Y epitope, whereas matching of the HLA-A2/H-Y epitope did not affect graft survival [5]. The prevalence of HLA-A1 male donors is 13% in the general German population. Consequently, global gender matching regardless of HLA restrictions did not have a significant effect on rejection-free graft survival [14]. These facts result in the recommendation that male HLA-A1-positive donors should not be allocated to female recipients.

1.3.1.2 HA-3

The HA-3 epitope is another HLA-A1-restricted H antigen that has been shown to be expressed in all corneal layers. This epitope is derived from the lymphoid blast crisis (Lbc) oncoprotein. Two alleles, VTEPGTAQY (HA-3T) and VMEPGTAQY (HA-3M) have been identified. T cell immune reactivity has only been observed in the direction of HA-3T. This constellation, however, was not associated with a statistically significantly increased incidence of graft rejections in a retrospective clinical investigation [5]. Furthermore, the prevalence of the immunogenic setting is as low as 3% in the German population. HLA-A1/HA-3 matching is thus not recommended for the clinical routine.

Table 1.1. A selection of human minor transplantation antigens

Name	Original gene	HLA restriction
HA-1	Histocompatibility (minor) HA-1	HLA-A2
HA-1/B60	Histocompatibility (minor) HA-1	HLA-B60
HA-2	Myosin IG	HLA-A2
HA-3	A kinase (PRKA) anchor protein 13	HLA-A1
HA-8	KIAA0020	HLA-A2
HB-1	Histocompatibility (minor) HB-1	HLA-B44
ACC-1	B-cell leukemia/lymphoma 2 related protein A1	HLA-A24
ACC-2	B-cell leukemia/lymphoma 2 related protein A1	HLA-B44
UGT2B17	UDP glucuronosyltransferase 2 family, polypeptide B17	HLA-A29
LRH-1	Purinergic receptor P2X, ligand-gated ion channel, 5	HLA-B7
SP110	SP110 nuclear body protein	HLA-A3
PANE1	Centromere protein M	HLA-A3
ECGF1	Endothelial cell growth factor 1 (platelet-derived)	HLA-B7
CTSH/A31	Cathepsin H	HLA-A31
CTSH/A33	Cathepsin H	HLA-A33
A2/HY	Smcy homolog, Y-linked	HLA-A2
B7/HY	Smcy homolog, Y-linked	HLA-B7
A1/HY	Ubiquitin specific peptidase 9, Y-linked	HLA-A1
B8/HY	Ubiquitously transcribed tetratricopeptide repeat gene, Y-linked	HLA-B8
B60/HY	Ubiquitously transcribed tetratricopeptide repeat gene, Y-linked	HLA-B60
DQ5/HY	DEAD (Asp-Glu-Ala-Asp) box polypeptide 3, Y-linked	HLA-DQ5
DR15/HY	DEAD (Asp-Glu-Ala-Asp) box polypeptide 3, Y-linked	HLA-DR15
B52/HY	Ribosomal protein S4, Y-linked 1	HLA-B52
DRB3*0301/HY	Ribosomal protein S4, Y-linked 1	HLA-DRB3*0301
A33/HY	Thymosin, beta 4, Y-linked	HLA-A33

1.3.1.3 ABO

A significant reduction in graft reactions from ABO (blood group) matching has been observed in high-risk penetrating keratoplasty, but not in normal-risk keratoplasties [6, 15, 23]. Additionally, a substantial proportion of failed corneal grafts seem to actually express ABO blood group antigens in the stroma and graft endothelial layers [1], where they are absent under physiological conditions. This finding suggests a direct immune response against mismatched ABO antigens. However, the beneficial effect from blood group matching might alternatively be ascribed to HLA-restricted H antigens originating from the ABO-specific glycosyl-transferases. Future research is needed to work out the exact mechanisms involved in blood group histocompatibility. In particular, finding the HLA restrictions of putative blood group H antigens might help when evaluating blood group matches for normal-risk situations, where the beneficial effects may only apply to a subgroup of patients.

Summary for the Clinician

- HLA-A1-positive grafts from male donors should not be allocated to female recipients
- Matching blood group antigens reduces graft rejections in high-risk keratoplasty
- The rapidly evolving field of minor antigens is the subject of ongoing and future research

1.4 Practical Concerns: Time on the Waiting List

1.4.1 Waiting Time Variability as a Major Handicap in HLA Matching

Histocompatibility matching is inevitably associated with additional time on the waiting list, since it entails refusing all newly available grafts until one that satisfies the histocompatibility requirements is identified. Due to the social and individual costs of blindness, waiting periods exceeding one year are barely reasonable.

The waiting period strongly depends on the recipient's histocompatibility antigens, and thus strongly varies inter-individually: patients with common HLA phenotypes can be routinely provided with a matching graft within a few months. This is intuitive, as the prevalence of compatible phenotypes is common in the donor population too. On the other hand, individuals with a rare HLA phenotype commonly remain on the waiting list for years without being allocated a compatible graft.

These patients in particular contribute to the reluctance to perform HLA matching that is currently prevalent in the clinical routine.

These patients could be spared waiting in vain for a long period if it was possible to identify them in advance. An alternative option would be to accept a few HLA mismatches, preferably of low immunogenicity (see Sect. 1.2.3). A method for predicting the waiting time is vital to the informed consent of the individual patient to histocompatibility.

1.4.2 Predicting the Time on the Waiting List

The prediction of time on the waiting list has to be based on the individual HLA phenotype, a database of haplotype frequencies in the donor population, and last but not least on parameters of the local cornea bank, such as the rate of newly available corneal grafts. This algorithm has been successfully validated with a historical waiting list of almost 1,400 HLA-typed patients [3] and is detailed in the following.

A maximum of 27 different HLA phenotypes match any recipient who is heterozygous at the HLA loci A, B and DR for combinatory reasons. In contrast, only one phenotype matches an individual who is completely homozygous. The total percentage of the donor population matching the HLA phenotype of any recipient is well approximated by the sum of all population frequencies (donor population) of the compatible HLA diplotypes. The frequency of any HLA diplotype is derived from the product of both of the respective haplotype frequencies. The haplotype frequencies of the HLA loci A, B and DR can be retrieved from a common database [21].

The daily rate of new HLA-compatible grafts is proportional to the daily rate of new HLA-typed grafts and the percentage of HLA compatible donors, as described above. Assuming a Poissonian distribution of donors, the expected waiting period is the reciprocal of the daily rate of new HLA-compatible grafts. These calculations have to be calibrated to the local cornea to yield actual waiting time estimations.

Summary for the Clinician

- Most patients can be served with an HLA-compatible graft well within a year, even when they are on a monocenter waiting list
- Patients that wait in vain for a HLA match for a long time contribute to the general reluctance to perform HLA matching in penetrating keratoplasty
- The waiting time for a histocompatible graft can be predicted from the HLA phenotype and discussed with the patient

1

1.5   Recommended Clinical Practice

All corneal grafts should be typed for at least the HLA loci A, B and DR. Molecular typing should be preferred over serologic methods, as molecular methods can still detect the HLA phenotype with excellent precision when blood samples are collected post mortem. An additional benefit of molecular typing is the applicability of the HLAMatchmaker algorithm (Sect. 1.2.3). Whenever possible, these data should be registered with supraregional allocation registries, such as Bio Implant Services (Leiden, The Netherlands), in order to build up a large pool for histocompatibility matching.

All potential graft recipients should also be typed, again preferably with immunogenetic techniques. All patients awaiting normal-risk keratoplasties should be confronted with their expected time on the waiting list. The improved prognosis resulting from HLA compatibility must be weighed against the expected waiting time. This strategy needs to be discussed with each patient individually.

Patients awaiting high-risk keratoplasty should be provided with a histocompatible graft (HLA and ABO) in almost all cases. The HLAMatchmaker algorithm can be applied to the balance time on the waiting list with the quality of histocompatibility that is realistically achievable.

Additional antigen systems (e.g., H-Y/HLA-A1 and ABO blood group antigens) should be accounted for by rejecting corneal grafts with strong immunologic potential in the individual setting.

In summary, long-term graft survival will most likely improve upon routinely matching major and certain minor histocompatibility antigens. An unpublished preliminary cost risk assessment indicates that HLA matching is cost-effective since the costs of HLA typing will be outweighed by the immune reactions avoided within a five-year horizon.

References

1. Ardjomand N, Komericki P, Klein A, Mattes D, El-Shabrawi Y, Radner H (2005) ABO blood group expression in corneal allograft failures. Ophthalmologe 102:981–986

2. Bartels MC, Doxiadis IIN, Colen TP, Beekhuis WH (2003) Long-term outcome in high-risk corneal transplantation and the influence of HLA-A and HLA-B matching. Cornea 22:552–556

3. Böhringer D, Reinhard T, Böhringer S, Enczmann J, Godehard E, Sundmacher R (2002) Predicting time on the waiting list for HLA matched corneal grafts. Tissue Antigens 59:407–411

4. Böhringer D, Reinhard T, Duquesnoy RJ, Böhringer S, Enczmann J, Lange P, Claas F, Sundmacher R (2004) Beneficial effect of matching at the HLA-A and -B amino-acid triplet level on rejection-free clear graft survival in penetrating keratoplasty. Transplantation 77:417–421

5. Böhringer D, Spierings E, Enczmann J, Bohringer S, Sundmacher R, Goulmy E, Reinhard T (2006) Matching of the minor histocompatibility antigen HLA-A1/H-Y may improve prognosis in corneal transplantation. Transplantation 82:1037–1041

6. Borderie VM, Lopez M, Vedie F, Laroche L (1997) ABO antigen blood-group compatibility in corneal transplantation. Cornea 16:1–6

7. Creemers PC, Kahn D, Hill JC (1999) HLA-A and -B alleles in cornea donors as risk factors for graft rejection. Transpl Immunol 7:15–18

8. Doxiadis II, Smits JM, Schreuder GM, Persijn GG, van Houwelingen HC, van Rood JJ, Claas FH (1996) Association between specific HLA combinations and probability of kidney allograft loss: the taboo concept. Lancet 348:850–853

9. Duquesnoy RJ (2002) HLAMatchmaker: a molecularly based algorithm for histocompatibility determination. I. Description of the algorithm. Hum Immunol 63:339–352

10. Duquesnoy RJ, Askar M (2007) HLAMatchmaker: a molecularly based algorithm for histocompatibility determination. V. Eplet matching for HLA-DR, HLA-DQ, and HLA-DP. Hum Immunol 68:12–25

11. Duquesnoy RJ, Takemoto S, de Lange P, Doxiadis IIN, Schreuder GMT, Persijn GG, Claas FHJ (2003) HLA matchmaker: a molecularly based algorithm for histocompatibility determination. III. Effect of matching at the HLA-A,B amino acid triplet level on kidney transplant survival. Transplantation 75:884–889

12. Haskova Z, Sproule TJ, Roopenian DC, Ksander, R B (2003) An immunodominant minor histocompatibility alloantigen that initiates corneal allograft rejection. Transplantation 75:1368–1374

13. Hopkins KA, Maguire MG, Fink NE, Bias WB (1992) Reproducibility of HLA-A, B, and DR typing using peripheral blood samples: results of retyping in the collaborative corneal transplantation studies. Collaborative Corneal Transplantation Studies Group (corrected). Hum Immunol 33:122–128

14. Inoue K, Amano S, Oshika T, Tsuru T (2000) Histocompatibility Y antigen compatibility and allograft rejection in corneal transplantation. Eye 14(Pt 2):201–205

15. Inoue K, Tsuru T (1999) ABO antigen blood-group compatibility and allograft rejection in corneal transplantation. Acta Ophthalmol Scand 77:495–499

16. Khaireddin R, Wachtlin J, Hopfenmuller W, Hoffmann F (2003) HLA-A, HLA-B and HLA-DR matching reduces

the rate of corneal allograft rejection. Graefes Arch Clin Exp Ophthalmol 241:1020–1028

17. Liu Y, Hamrah P, Zhang Q, Taylor AW, Dana MR (2002) Draining lymph nodes of corneal transplant hosts exhibit evidence for donor major histocompatibility complex (MHC) class II-positive dendritic cells derived from MHC class II-negative grafts. J Exp Med 195:259–268

18. Reinhard T, Böhringer D, Enczmann J, Kogler G, Mayweg S, Wernet P, Sundmacher R (2004) Improvement of graft prognosis in penetrating normal-risk keratoplasty by HLA class I and II matching. Eye 18:269–277

19. Reinhard T, Reis A, Böhringer D, Malinowski M, Voiculescu A, Heering P, Godehardt E, Sundmacher R (2001) Systemic mycophenolate mofetil in comparison with systemic cyclosporin A in high-risk keratoplasty patients: 3 years' results of a randomized prospective clinical trial. Graefes Arch Clin Exp Ophthalmol 239:367–372

20. Reinhard T, Spelsberg H, Henke L, Kontopoulos T, Enczmann J, Wernet P, Berschick P, Sundmacher R, Böhringer D (2004) Long-term results of allogeneic penetrating limbo-keratoplasty in total limbal stem cell deficiency. Ophthalmology 111:775–782

21. Schipper RF, Oudshoorn M, D'Amaro J, van der Zanden HG, de Lange P, Bakker JT, Bakker J, van Rood JJ (1996) Validation of large data sets, an essential prerequisite for data analysis: an analytical survey of the bone marrow donors worldwide. Tissue Antigens 47:169–178

22. Spierings E, Wieles B, Goulmy E (2004) Minor histocompatibility antigens—big in tumour therapy. Trends Immunol 25:56–60

23. The Collaborative Corneal Transplantation Studies Research Group (1992) The collaborative corneal transplantation studies (CCTS). Effectiveness of histocompatibility matching in high-risk corneal transplantation. Arch Ophthalmol 110:1392–1403

24. Völker-Dieben HJ, Claas FH, Schreuder GM, Schipper RF, Pels E, Persijn GG, Smits J, D'Amaro J (2000) Beneficial effect of HLA-DR matching on the survival of corneal allografts. Transplantation 70:640–648

25. Yamada J, Streilein JW (1998) Fate of orthotopic corneal allografts in C57BL/6 mice. Transpl Immunol 6:161–168

Chapter 2

Acute Anterior Uveitis and HLA-B27: What's New?

2

John H. Chang, Peter J. McCluskey, Denis Wakefield

Core Messages

- Acute anterior uveitis (AAU) accounts for 90% of all uveitis cases seen by the general ophthalmologist.
- About half of all AAU cases are HLA-B27-associated.
- HLA-B27+ AAU represents a distinct clinical entity with important ocular and extraocular consequences.
- The typical ocular phenotype of HLA-B27+ AAU is that of acute onset, unilateral inflammation of the iris and ciliary body, with a tendency towards recurrent attacks and more severe inflammation, including hypopyon formation. Males are affected more frequently than females.
- All patients with AAU must have a dilated fundus examination to confirm the diagnosis is anterior uveitis, and careful clinical assessment regarding possible associated systemic inflammatory disease.
- All patients with AAU should be investigated with HLA-B27 typing, syphilis serology, and a chest X-ray at a minimum.

- 50% of patients with HLA-B27+ AAU will develop an associated seronegative spondyloarthropathy (SpA), whilst approximately 25% of the patients initially diagnosed with HLA-B27-associated systemic disease will develop AAU.
- HLA-B27 is the strongest known genetic risk factor for AAU. There are multiple subtypes of HLA-B27, which may be differentially associated with disease.
- In addition to genetic factors, environmental factors play a critical role in the pathogenesis of AAU.
- Bacterial triggers have been strongly implicated in the development of AAU and recurrent episodes of ocular inflammation.
- Human uveal antigen-presenting cells express TLR4, the receptor for LPS, and may provide a critical molecular link between microbial triggers and the development of AAU.
- Topical corticosteroids and cycloplegic agents are the mainstay of treatment.

2.1 Introduction

Acute anterior uveitis (AAU) is by far the most common form of uveitis [6]. It is characterized by a breakdown in the blood–aqueous barrier and acute inflammation of the iris and ciliary body. Immunopathologically, there is up-regulation of cell adhesion molecules on the uveal vasculature and aqueous humor expression of pro-inflammatory cytokines such as tumor necrosis factor (TNF)-α, interferon (IFN)-γ and chemokines that selectively recruit and activate inflammatory cells (neutrophils, monocytes and lymphocytes) into the uvea and anterior chamber (AC). These cells are visible clinically on slit lamp biomicroscopy. The breakdown in the blood–ocular barrier results in leakage of serum proteins from the uveal vasculature into the AC, which is visible on biomicroscopy as aqueous flare and fibrin formation. Keratic precipitates (KPs) represent inflammatory cells that have precipitated on the corneal endothelium. Thus AAU is a prototypical inflammatory disease in which the clinician is uniquely able to visualize the inflammatory response in vivo and all of its sequelae using the slit lamp biomicroscope, and to correlate it with the immunopathological process.

About 50% of all cases of AAU are associated with the presence of HLA-B27, a class I major histocompatibility complex (MHC) [8]. HLA-B27-associated AAU represents a distinct clinical phenotype that may be associated with severe intraocular inflammation as well as systemic inflammatory diseases such as the seronegative spondyloarthropathies (SpA). There has been some recent

2

progress in our understanding of the clinical features and the immunopathogenesis of this group of diseases. The aim of the present chapter is to highlight these advances for the clinician managing patients suffering from AAU.

2.2 Epidemiology of Acute Anterior Uveitis and HLA-B27

The annual incidence of uveitis has been reported to be between 17 and 52 per 100,000 population, with a prevalence of between 38 and 714 per 100,000 population [6]. Anterior uveitis is the predominant form of uveitis in most populations studied, accounting for approximately 50–60% of all cases of uveitis seen in tertiary referral centers. In the general community, AAU accounts for up to 90% of all uveitis cases once referral study bias has been removed [22]. In one study, the mean annual incidence and prevalence rates of anterior uveitis were, respectively, 21 and 69 per 100,000 population, whilst the total incidence and prevalence rates of all cases of uveitis in that community were 23 and 75 per 100,000 population, respectively [29].

HLA-B27-associated AAU is the most important form of anterior uveitis (acute and chronic forms combined), accounting for 18–32% of all cases of anterior uveitis (see Table 2.1 for common causes of acute and chronic

anterior uveitis). As will be discussed later, HLA-B27 is the strongest known genetic risk factor for AAU. The lifetime cumulative incidence of AAU in the general population has been reported to be about 0.2%, but this increases to 1% in the HLA-B27-positive population [19].

HLA-B27+ AAU demonstrates a clear gender preponderance, with males being about 2.5 times more likely to be affected than females. The first attack of HLA-B27+ AAU occurs between 20 and 40 years of age in the great majority of cases, and these patients are about a decade younger than their HLA-B27 negative counterparts at the time of disease onset [8].

2.2.1 Global Patterns of HLA-B27+ Acute Anterior Uveitis

In the general Caucasian population, the prevalence of HLA-B27 is approximately 8%, whereas the HLA-B27 antigen is present in about half of the patients suffering from AAU [8]. There is a global variation in the prevalence of the HLA-B27 gene, and due to this, as well as potential variations in other genetic and environmental factors that are relevant to disease pathogenesis; there are distinct global patterns of AAU. For example, the relatively lower frequency of HLA-B27+ AAU in Asia reflects the lower prevalence of HLA-B27 in this area; it is as low as 0.5% in Japan [6, 8].

Table 2.1. Common causes of acute and chronic anterior uveitis

Acute anterior uveitis (AAU)	Chronic anterior uveitis
HLA-B27+ AAU	Juvenile idiopathic arthritis (JIA)
Ocular involvement only	
Ankylosing spondylitis	
Reactive arthritis	
Psoriatic arthropathy	
Inflammatory bowel disease	
Undifferentiated SpA	
Idiopathic AAU (HLA-B27 negative)	Fuch's heterochromic iridocyclitis
Sarcoid uveitis	Idiopathic
Behçet's disease	Sarcoid uveitis
Posner–Schlossman Syndrome	Syphilitic uveitis
Lens-associated uveitis	Herpetic (herpes zoster/simplex)
Syphilitic uveitis	

Summary for the Clinician

- ■ AAU is the most common form (90%) of uveitis
- ■ Approximately half of all patients with AAU are positive for HLA-B27
- ■ There are global variations in the prevalence of HLA-B27 AAU
- ■ HLA-B27 AAU represents a distinct clinical entity with clinically important ocular and extraocular implications
- ■ Males are affected about 2.5 times more frequently with HLA-B27 AAU than females
- ■ First attack of HLA-B27 AAU usually occurs between 20 and 40 years of age

2.3 HLA-B27 and Disease

HLA-B27 is a human leukocyte antigen (HLA) class I molecule whose strong associations with disease set it apart from most HLA antigens, and so it has been the subject of much research over the past 35 years. HLA molecules are encoded on the short arm of chromosome 6. HLA antigens are vital to normal immune surveillance and the generation of immune responses to foreign antigens. These molecules are critically important in various physiologic and pathologic immune processes, including antiviral responses, organ transplantation immunology and tumor immunology, and play a key role in the pathogenesis of an expanding list of immune-mediated inflammatory diseases. HLA antigens are divided into HLA class I and class II molecules, which have distinct structural and functional characteristics (Table 2.2). HLA molecules present antigenic peptides to T lymphocytes via distinct antigen processing and HLA-restricted presentation pathways, with the common goal of initiating the antigen-specific adaptive immune response.

Table 2.2. HLA class I and class II molecules

	HLA class I	HLA class II
Subclass	HLA-A, -B, -C (classical)	HLA-DR, -DQ, -DP
	HLA-E, -F, -G (non-classical)	
Cellular expression	Most human somatic cells	Antigen-presenting cells
	No/minimal expression on uveal or corneal endothelial cells	Dendritic cells
		Macrophages
		Monocytes
Antigen (Ag) presented	Endogenous or intracellular peptides (self or viral origin)	Exogenous or extracellular peptides
T cell presentation	Presents Ag to CD8+ (cytotoxic) T lymphocytes	Presents Ag to CD4+ (helper) T cells
Examples of well-known disease associations	HLA-B27 and AAU, AS.	HLA-DR, -DQ subtypes and VKHD
	HLA-29 and birdshot retinochoroidopathy	HLA-DR15 and pars planitis
	HLA-B51 and Behçet's disease	HLA-DR4 and sympathetic ophthalmia

AAU, Acute anterior uveitis; *AS*, ankylosing spondylitis; *VKHD*, Vogt–Koyanagi–Harada disease

The strong association between HLA-B27 and inflammatory diseases, such as ankylosing spondylitis (AS), reactive arthritis (including Reiter's syndrome) and AAU has been known for over 30 years [2, 3, 8]. Within this spectrum of HLA-B27-associated inflammatory diseases, AS demonstrates the strongest association, with around 90% of patients possessing the HLA-B27 antigen. Nearly a third of these patients develop HLA-B27+ AAU during the clinical course of their extraocular inflammatory disease. Despite extensive research for other genes, HLA-B27 is still the strongest known genetic risk factor for the development of AAU, but how it predisposes to disease remains an enigma. Possession of the HLA-B27 antigen increases the relative risk of AAU by 26 times [3]. Although 45–70% of patients with AAU are HLA-B27 positive compared to only 4–8% of the general Caucasian population, it should be appreciated that 99% of subjects that have the HLA-B27 gene are healthy and will not develop associated diseases during their lifetime. This implies that other genetic factors and environmental factors such as microbial triggers play an important role in the development of AAU (as discussed in Sect. 2.3.2).

X ray crystallography has demonstrated the three-dimensional structure of HLA-B27. It is a heterodimeric membrane-bound glycoprotein consisting of a polymorphic α chain, which is noncovalently linked to non polymorphic β-2-microglobulin. The α chains contain two peptide-binding domains (α1 and α2) which form antigen-binding clefts that bind short peptides of 8–12 amino acids [20].

2.3.1   New Developments in the Immunogenetics of HLA-B27

Recent studies have shown that HLA-B27 is not a single allele but a family of at least 31 different alleles that encode for HLA-B27 subtypes (named HLA-B*2701 to HLA-B*2728) [17]. There is a varied distribution of these HLA-B27 subtypes in different populations, and this may account for the varying strengths of HLA-B27-disease association that are observed in different ethnic groups. The more common subtypes, HLA-B*2705 (accounts for about 90% of HLA-B27+ individuals of northern European descent), B*2702 and B*2704, have been shown to be strongly associated with AS [17]. Both HLA-B*2705 and B*2702 were also strongly associated with AAU in a study of Dutch patients [11]. There has not been a study of other HLA-B27 subtypes and their association with AAU. However, at least two subtypes, HLA-B*2706 (common in Southeast Asia) and B*2709

2

(found in Sardinia) appear to lack a disease association with AS [17]. These HLA-B27 subtypes vary from each other by only one or several amino acids, mostly at the antigen-binding region of the molecule, and are thus expected to alter the range of antigenic peptides bound and presented to T cells by HLA-B27. The finding of differential HLA-B27 subtype disease association thus suggests that the antigen-presentation function of HLA-B27 may play an important role in the pathogenesis of disease. Such observations support the "arthritogenic" or "uveitogenic" peptide hypothesis for AS or HLA-B27+ AAU pathogenesis, which proposes that disease is a consequence of self-reactive cytotoxic T lymphocytes (via molecular mimicry) that are activated against a peptide found only in the joint or uvea [8, 17].

Recent studies using animal models of HLA-B27-associated inflammatory diseases have clearly demonstrated the direct pathogenic role of HLA-B27. HLA-B27 transgenic rats and mice that express human HLA-B27 antigens were found to spontaneously develop a multisystemic inflammatory disease resembling the spectrum of human HLA-B27-associated spondyloarthropathies (SpA) [8, 18, 31]. Of particular interest, these transgenic animals were healthy if kept in a germ-free environment, but once moved to a normal environment and exposed to commensal microbes, acute development of enterocolitis, ankylosing arthritis, enthesitis, psoriasiform skin lesions and inflammatory male genital lesions were triggered [32]. This provides further evidence to support not only the importance of genetic factors but that of environmental factors and in particular, microbial triggers, in the development of HLA-B27-associated diseases (see the next section). Interestingly, however, AAU was not a prominent feature of the HLA-B27 transgenic animal models.

Summary for the Clinician

■ Although other genes are almost certainly involved, HLA-B27 remains the strongest known genetic risk factor for AAU.
■ HLA-B27 is not a single allele. Instead, there are multiple subtypes of HLA-B27, which appear to have differential associations with disease. The more common subtypes, HLA-B*2705, B*2702 and B*2704, are strongly associated with AS and AAU.
■ Transgenic animals expressing human HLA-B27 spontaneously develop a multisystemic inflammatory disease.

2.3.2 Role of Microbial Triggers in Immune-Mediated Inflammation

It is clear that specific environmental factors play a critical role in the development of HLA-B27 AAU, as the great majority of HLA-B27-positive individuals do not develop inflammatory diseases despite the strong relative genetic risk of developing AS or AAU. In particular, there is extensive evidence from both clinical and experimental studies that support the role of microbial triggers in the development of AAU. Reactive arthritis and uveitis are prototypical examples of the development of noninfectious immune-mediated inflammation following a triggering genitourinary or gastrointestinal tract infection. *Chlamydia trachomatis* and Gram-negative bacteria, such as certain species of *Salmonella, Shigella, Campylobacter, Klebsiella* and *Yersinia*, have been implicated in the pathogenesis of HLA-B27+ AAU [8]. The precise pathogenic mechanism remains unclear, but putative "uveitogenic" peptides from these bacteria have been shown to have the necessary sequences to be able to be bound and presented by HLA-B27 to T cells. It has been proposed that these microbe-derived antigens may trigger CD8+ T cell immune responses that cross-react with self-tissue antigens (molecular mimicry) that are uniquely found in the uvea or joint tissue, resulting in auto-immune tissue inflammation [8].

Microbial triggers have been implicated in the pathogenesis of recurrent attacks of HLA-B27+ AAU. Raised antibody levels against *Salmonella, Campylobacter jejuni, Klebsiella pneumonia* and *Yersinia* were found to be associated with recurrent attacks of AAU [15]. Furthermore, a close relation between the recurrences of AAU and chronic asymptomatic ileocolitis has been observed, implicating a pathogenic role for mucosal infection in the development of anterior uveitis [1].

It is also of interest that many animal models of anterior uveitis involve the induction of ocular inflammation with microbial cell wall components, such as endotoxin or lipopolysaccharide (LPS) of Gram-negative bacteria, and peptidoglycan (PGN) or lipoteichoic acid (LTA) of Gram-positive bacteria [8, 9]. The eye appears to be highly and selectively sensitive to the pro-inflammatory effects of LPS in endotoxin-induced uveitis (EIU), with no significant abnormalities observed in other organs in response to the uveitogenic dose of LPS. EIU is the most widely used animal model for AAU, and a low dose of LPS given at a site remote from the eye induces an acute breakdown in the blood–aqueous barrier and the influx of acute inflammatory cells into the anterior uvea and AC [8, 26]. Some of the recent developments in our understanding of innate immunity and the Toll-like receptors (TLR) have led to new insights into the potential mechanisms behind these important observations linking microbial triggers and inflammatory disease, including AAU (see Sect. 2.5.2) [9].

2.3.3   HLA-B27-Associated Inflammatory Disease

HLA-B27 is associated with not just AAU but a spectrum of seronegative spondyloarthropathies (SpA). The strongest disease association of HLA-B27 is with ankylosing spondylitis (AS), but the other HLA-B27-associated inflammatory diseases include reactive arthritis, inflammatory bowel disease (IBD) and its associated arthropathy, psoriatic arthropathy, and undifferentiated SpA. From the available data, it is estimated that more than half of the patients with HLA-B27+ AAU will develop AS or one of the other SpA, whilst approximately 25% of the patients initially diagnosed with HLA-B27 associated systemic disease will develop AAU during their lifetime [8]. The ophthalmologist must be aware of these systemic disease associations of HLA-B27 AAU, as he is uniquely placed to recognize a unifying systemic HLA-B27-related diagnosis in patients with AAU and symptoms of joint, skin or GIT dysfunction. This requires careful clinical assessment, follow-up and referral to the relevant internist for further investigation.

2.4   Other Genetic Risk Factors for Acute Anterior Uveitis

Observations, including those from twin concordance studies and of familial aggregation of AAU, indicate that there are other non-HLA-B27 genes, both within and outside the MHC, that predispose to the development of AAU. HLA-B27-positive first-degree relatives of patients with HLA-B27 AAU have a higher risk (13%) of developing AAU than HLA-B27-positive individuals without affected relatives (1%) [12]. Recent genome-wide scans of families with multiple affected members with AAU have identified several chromosomal regions associated with AAU, including regions on chromosomes 3, 5, 9, 13 and 15. Strong linkage was observed at a locus at chromosome 9p21–9p24 that uniquely associated with AAU but not with AS [21].

Chemokines play a pathogenic role in AAU by recruiting inflammatory cells to the AC (see Sect. 2.5.1). A recent study has reported a significantly increased frequency of a functional polymorphism in the promoter region of the gene for the chemokine CCL2/monocyte chemoattractant protein (MCP)-1 in patients with HLA-B27+ AAU compared to HLA-B27+ healthy controls [35].

Similarly, there are also probably as-yet-unidentified genetic risk factors for idiopathic HLA-B27-negative AAU. For example, MHC class I chain-associated gene A (MICA) A4 allele was found to be at significantly higher frequency in patients with HLA-B27-negative AAU compared to that in ethnically matched HLA-B27-negative controls [14].

2.5   Current Understanding of AAU Pathogenesis

There have been recent advances in our understanding of the immunopathogenesis of AAU due to the existence of several good animal models of AAU, as well as the development of powerful new research tools, such as intravital microscopy for studying leukocyte interactions with the uveal vasculature in vivo during the various stages of experimental AAU, advances in molecular biology (such as DNA microarrays that can rapidly screen for tens of thousands of genes), and advances in proteomics. However, although we are now able to dissect the multitude of molecular steps in the evolution of acute intraocular inflammation and the individual effects of modulating these pathways, there is still much to be learned. For example, the critical initial processes involved in the breakdown of ocular immune privilege, the restriction of inflammation to one eye, the triggering of recurrent attacks of AAU, or the processes responsible for the progression of AAU

Summary for the Clinician

- Environmental factors, in particular microbial triggers, are clearly important in the pathogenesis of AAU.
- *Chlamydia trachomatis* and Gram-negative bacteria have been implicated in the pathogenesis of HLA-B27+ AAU, including certain species of *Salmonella, Shigella, Campylobacter, Klebsiella* and *Yersinia*.
- Microbial products, such as LPS of Gram-negative bacteria, have been used to induce various animal models of AAU. The most widely adopted model of AAU is endotoxin-induced uveitis (EIU).
- Patients with HLA-B27 AAU are at increased risk of developing an associated systemic inflammatory disease, and vice versa.

to chronic inflammation are unknown. The elucidation of these immune mechanisms may lead to the development of truly revolutionary therapies for halting AAU early and preventing the development of sight-threatening, recurrent or chronic anterior uveitis.

2.5.1 Cytokines

Cytokines are soluble mediators produced by various cells of the innate and adaptive immune system that orchestrate, coordinate and integrate these two arms of the immune response. Cytokines typically have pleiotropic effects, including pro-inflammatory, anti-inflammatory and chemoattractant functions. Leukocyte extravasation from the blood into the tissue is a regulated multistep process involving a series of coordinated interactions between leukocytes and endothelial cells involving selectin-mediated rolling, integrin-mediated firm adhesion, and chemokine-mediated migration. Chemokines are of pathogenic importance in the selective intraocular recruitment of neutrophils, monocytes and CD4+ T lymphocytes in uveitis.

Each step of the cell recruitment process is important in the pathogenesis of experimental AAU, and selectively inhibiting any step will partially abrogate uveal inflammation. There is significant redundancy in the process, with another pro-inflammatory pathway being able to largely take over the role of one that has been selectively inhibited.

High aqueous humor levels of various pro-inflammatory cytokines, such as TNF-γ, IFN-γ, IL-2 and IL-12, and low intraocular expression of the anti-inflammatory cytokine IL-10 have been shown in human AAU [8]. Elevated aqueous humor expression of chemokines that selectively recruit the acute inflammatory cells in AAU have been demonstrated in patients with active AAU. IL-8/CXCL8 (recruits neutrophils), interferon-gamma-inducible protein (IP)-10/CXCL10, MCP-1/CCL2, RANTES (regulated upon activation, normal T cell expressed and secreted)/CCL5 and macrophage inflammatory protein (MIP)-1β/CCL4 (recruits monocytes and activated T cells) were significantly elevated during the active stages of AAU and correlated with the clinical severity of the disease [34].

2.5.2 Toll-Like Receptors (TLR)

Recent progress in our knowledge of a family of innate immune receptors called Toll-like receptors (TLRs) has shed new light on our understanding of the normal host immune defense against microbes and the pathogenesis of a wide range of infectious and noninfectious autoimmune diseases. TLRs are a family of so-called pattern recognition receptors (PRR) that recognize "signature patterns" of microbes called "pathogen-associated molecular patterns" (PAMPs). Ten human TLRs have been identified to date, each of which recognize PAMPs from a unique class of microbes; for example, TLR4 responds to LPS of Gram-negative bacterial cell wall whilst TLR2 recognizes Gram-positive bacterial cell wall components [9, 23, 30]. Thus, the discovery of TLRs has conferred a degree of specificity to innate immunity that had not been previously recognized [23]. Activation of TLRs by their ligands results in the initiation of a pro-inflammatory cascade, the activation of the transcription factor NFκB, leading to the production of pro-inflammatory cytokines, chemokines and activation of immune cells. Thus, these PRRs allow the innate immune system to respond rapidly to microbes at host/environment interfaces that express high levels of TLRs [9, 30]. There has been immense research on this family of receptors in the past decade, and they have since been implicated in the pathogenesis of a variety of inflammatory diseases, including IBD, AS and psoriasis [5, 30, 36]. Notably, all of these diseases can be complicated by AAU and are recognized systemic associations with HLA-B27+ AAU. In IBD, it is thought that inappropriate and hyper-responsive inflammation triggered by various TLRs to commensal gut bacteria may play a critical role in the observed chronic intestinal inflammation.

Functional TLR4 expression by uveal antigen-presenting cells (APC) in the normal human iris and ciliary body has been recently demonstrated [4, 7, 9]. This provides a novel mechanism by which the various implicated microbial triggers could initiate the development of AAU, and explains the apparent high sensitivity of the uvea to LPS (now recognized as being the ligand for TLR4). LPS activation of perivascular TLR4-expressing uveal dendritic cells (DCs) could lead to the production of pro-inflammatory cytokines and the activation of vascular adhesion molecules, a breakdown in the blood–ocular barrier, and the recruitment of inflammatory cells to the AC [7, 9]. TLR4 is absolutely essential for inflammatory responses to LPS. In the animal model for AAU, the C3H/HeN strain of mice (which are highly sensitive to developing EIU) has normal functional TLR4, whilst the congenic C3H/HeJ strain with nonfunctional TLR4 does not develop EIU [9, 30].

Perturbations in the expression and function of TLR4 and TLR2 have been observed in patients with active AAU, further supporting the potential pathogenic role of these PRRs in the development of AAU [10]. These TLRs could provide the missing molecular link between the observations of microbial triggers and the development of AAU and other immune-mediated inflammatory disorders, but further studies are still required.

Summary for the Clinician

- Increased levels of pro-inflammatory cytokines and chemokines are found in the aqueous humor of patients with active AAU
- Toll-like receptors (TLR) are a family of pattern recognition receptors that recognize a variety of microbial products and lead to inflammation
- TLRs have been implicated in the pathogenesis of numerous inflammatory diseases, including HLA-B27-associated AS, IBD and AAU
- EIU, the animal model for AAU, is critically dependent on functional TLR4, the receptor for LPS of Gram-negative bacteria
- Uveal APCs in the human eye express TLR4, and perturbations in the TLRs have been observed in patients with AAU

Table 2.3. Standardized (SUN[a]) grading system for AC cell and flare severity [30]

Grade	AC cells	AC flare
0	None	None
0.5+	1–5 cells in the field[b]	-
1+	6–15 cells[b]	Faint
2+	16–25 cells[b]	Moderate (iris and lens details are clear)
3+	26–50 cells[b]	Marked (iris and lens details are hazy)
4+	>50 cells[b]	Intense (fibrin or plasmoid aqueous)

[a]Standardization of Uveitis Nomenclature (SUN)
[b]Field size used is a 1 mm by 1 mm slit beam. The presence or absence of a hypopyon should be noted separately in addition to the AC cellular activity grade

2.6   Clinical Features of Acute Anterior Uveitis

2.6.1   HLA-B27 and Clinical Phenotype

AAU presents with the clinical features of acute inflammation in the anterior segment of the eye (primarily the iris, ciliary body and AC). The typical phenotype of HLA-B27-positive AAU is that of abrupt onset of unilateral, often alternating, nongranulomatous AAU, characterized by the acute onset of a red, photophobic, painful eye and significant cellular and protein extravasation into the aqueous humor, clinically detectable as AC cells and flare on slit lamp examination. There is a standardized international grading system for grading AC cells and flare activity (Table 2.3, Standardization of Uveitis Nomenclature) [16]. HLA-B27-positive AAU has a high tendency to recur, and shows a significant association with other HLA-B27-related systemic diseases [8]. An episode lasts 6–8 weeks on average, and in cases of recurrent AAU, the intervals between the recurrent attacks are highly variable (from months to years).

In contrast, HLA-B27-negative anterior uveitis tends to be a more heterogeneous entity that is more likely to become bilateral or chronic uveitis, and which is infrequently associated with systemic diseases. Recurrent inflammation is not uncommon in HLA-B27-negative

AAU [8]. There is a subset of idiopathic HLA-B27-negative AAU that is clinically difficult to distinguish from HLA-B27-positive AAU.

2.6.2   Ocular Complications

Although AAU is generally associated with a good visual prognosis, it is not without its complications or visual morbidity, especially with recurrent attacks of ocular inflammation. In a study on the causes of visual impairment and blindness in intraocular inflammatory diseases, 10% of patients with HLA-B27-associated anterior uveitis suffered legal blindness or severe visual impairment [28]. Another case series found that 7% of their 175 patients with HLA-B27-associated uveitis demonstrated significantly decreased final visual acuity (>2 Snellen lines) [24]. The most important cause of reduced vision in patients with AAU is cystoid macular edema (CME), which has been reported to be as high as 17–25% [8, 24, 25], although these figures are almost certainly higher than those seen in the community, due to the influence of referral bias in these studies.

Posterior synechiae is by far the commonest complication of AAU. With the development of recurrent AAU or chronic inflammation, cataract and secondary glaucoma (as complications of the inflammation itself or induced by corticosteroid therapy) frequently cause visual impairment. Complications in patients with HLA-B27 related AAU are related to the number of recurrent attacks [27, 33].

2

Summary for the Clinician

- HLA-B27-positive AAU exhibits a distinct clinical phenotype compared to its HLA-B27 negative counterpart. This includes a tendency for recurrent attacks of inflammation, increased tendency for more severe AC inflammation including fibrinous reaction and hypopyon formation, and significant associations with extraocular inflammatory disease.
- There is a new international grading system for AC inflammatory activity (the Standardized Uveitis Nomenclature).
- About 10% of patients with HLA-B27-associated anterior uveitis suffer significant visual impairment due to sight-threatening complications such as CME, cataracts and secondary glaucoma.

2.7 Clinical Management of AAU

The investigation of AAU should be governed by the clinical history, the review of systems, and examination findings. In particular, careful attention should be paid to symptoms of possible associated systemic diseases, such as inflammatory back pain of AS, skin changes of psoriasis, or gastrointestinal symptoms of IBD. Dilated fundus examination is mandatory in the assessment of any patient with "anterior uveitis," in order to ensure that the disease is confined to the anterior segment and that the symptomatic anterior uveitis is not part of an intermediate or panuveitis.

There is no consensus on the extent of investigations indicated for the first episode of AAU. We recommend HLA-B27 typing, a chest X ray and syphilis serology as the minimum investigations for patients with their first attack of AAU. The HLA-B27 status has significant implications regarding the potential risk of further recurrent episode(s) of AAU (often a primary concern for the patient suffering their first attack) and the risk of developing HLA-B27 associated SpA. Syphilis serology remains a cost-effective investigation for syphilis, an increasingly common, treatable infectious cause of all forms of uveitis, including AAU [13]. A chest X-ray is recognized as being a useful screening investigation for asymptomatic pulmonary sarcoidosis, which may present as acute uveitis.

The mainstay of AAU treatment consists of topical corticosteroids, the intensity of administration of which is tailored to the severity of the AC inflammation. The general principle is to hit the inflammation hard early on in its course with intensive topical steroids, such as with prednisolone acetate 1% drops hourly initially. More severe inflammation associated with fibrin formation, hypopyon or severe pain may require subconjunctival steroid therapy or oral corticosteroids. Topical cycloplegic agents, such as atropine or homatropine, are essential for minimizing posterior synechiae formation and providing symptomatic relief from pain and photophobia. Topical steroids are slowly tapered over 6–8 weeks once the inflammatory activity is controlled. The total treatment course should cover at least 6–8 weeks to minimize premature cessation of topical steroids, which would be associated with a relapse in the partially treated inflammation (rather than a true recurrence) and would ultimately prolong the overall treatment course and increase the risk of developing chronic uveitis.

Systemic treatment with corticosteroids may be required to treat very severe uveitis that is resistant to maximum topical and local corticosteroid therapy. Other immunosuppressive agents are rarely needed to manage patients with recurrent AAU. Drugs such as salazopyrine and methotrexate are commonly used to treat IBD and SpA, and anecdotally there is evidence that this may decrease the frequency and severity of attacks of AAU. Chronic anterior uveitis associated with CME and reduced vision may, in selected patients, benefit from systemic immunosuppressive therapy. Exciting new biologic treatment modalities are being evaluated, including anti-TNFα therapy, anti-VEGF (vascular endothelial growth factor) therapy, and HLA-B27 peptide oral tolerance [8]. However, there is insufficient evidence to support the use of these newer agents at present, and more studies are required to establish their clinical indications, efficacy and safety.

2.8 Conclusions

AAU is a common condition that affects relatively young patients and can cause significant distress to the patient, with recurrent, unpredictable attacks of acute inflammation. Furthermore, AAU can be associated with sight-threatening complications such as CMO, and therefore it represents an important cause of visual impairment. The unique association between HLA-B27 AAU and its related systemic inflammatory diseases demands a comprehensive and holistic approach to managing patients with AAU, often requiring careful follow-up and liaison between multiple specialists. The great majority of uveitis cases seen by the general ophthalmologist will be AAU, and about half of these will be HLA-B27+ AAU, thus highlighting their clinical importance. Recent advances in our understanding of the genetics, immunology and pathogenesis of this condition will hopefully lead to improved care of our patients suffering from AAU.

References

1. Banares AA, Jover JA, Fernandez-Gutierrez B, et al. (1995) Bowel inflammation in anterior uveitis and spondyloarthropathy. J Rheumatol 22:1112–1117
2. Brewerton DA, Hart FD, Nicholls A, Caffrey M, James DC, Sturrock RD (1973) Ankylosing spondylitis and HL-A 27. Lancet 1:904–907
3. Brewerton DA, Caffrey M, Nicholls A, Walters D, James DC (1973) Acute anterior uveitis and HL-A 27. Lancet 2:994–996
4. Brito BE, Zamora DO, Bonnah RA, Pan Y, Planck SR, Rosenbaum JT (2004) Toll-like receptor 4 and CD14 expression in human ciliary body and TLR-4 in human iris endothelial cells. Exp Eye Res 79:203–208
5. Cario E, Podolsky DK (2000) Differential alteration in intestinal epithelial cell expression of toll-like receptor 3 (TLR3) and TLR4 in inflammatory bowel disease. Infect Immun 68:7010–7017
6. Chang JH, Wakefield D (2002) Uveitis: a global perspective. Ocular Immunol Inflamm 10:263–279
7. Chang JH, McCluskey P, Wakefield D (2004) Expression of toll-like receptor 4 and its associated lipopolysaccharide receptor complex by resident antigen-presenting cells in the human uvea. Invest Ophthalmol Vis Sci 45:1871–1878
8. Chang JH, McCluskey PJ, Wakefield D (2005) Acute anterior uveitis and HLA-B27. Surv Ophthalmol 50:364–388
9. Chang JH, McCluskey PJ, Wakefield D (2006) Toll-like receptors in ocular immunity and the immunopathogenesis of inflammatory eye disease. Br J Ophthalmol 90:103–108
10. Chang JH, Hampartzoumian T, Everett B, Lloyd A, McCluskey PJ, Wakefield D (2007) Changes in Toll-like receptor (TLR)-2 and TLR4 expression and function but not polymorphisms are associated with acute anterior uveitis. Invest Ophthalmol Vis Sci 48:1711–1717
11. Derhaag PJ, de Waal LP, Linssen A, Feltkamp TE (1988) Acute anterior uveitis and HLA-B27 subtypes. Invest Ophthalmol Visual Sci 29:1137–1140
12. Derhaag PJ, Linssen A, Broekema N, de Waal LP, Feltkamp TE (1988) A familial study of the inheritance of HLA-B27-positive acute anterior uveitis. Am J Ophthalmol 105:603–606
13. Doris JP, Saha K, Jones NP, Sukthankar A (2006) Ocular syphilis: the new epidemic. Eye (London, England) 20:703–705
14. Goto K, Ota M, Maksymowych WP, et al. (1998) Association between MICA gene A4 allele and acute anterior uveitis in white patients with and without HLA-B27. Am J Ophthalmol 126:436–441
15. Huhtinen M, Laasila K, Granfors K, et al. (2002) Infectious background of patients with a history of acute anterior uveitis. Ann Rheumatic Dis 61:1012–1016
16. Jabs DA, Nussenblatt RB, Rosenbaum JT (2005) Standardization of uveitis nomenclature for reporting clinical data. Results of the First International Workshop. Am J Ophthalmol 140:509–516
17. Khan MA, Mathieu A, Sorrentino R, Akkoc N (2007) The pathogenetic role of HLA-B27 and its subtypes. Autoimmun Rev 6:183–189
18. Khare SD, Luthra HS, David CS (1995) Spontaneous inflammatory arthritis in HLA-B27 transgenic mice lacking beta 2-microglobulin: a model of human spondyloarthropathies. J Exp Med 182:1153–1158
19. Linssen A, Rothova A, Valkenburg HA, et al. (1991) The lifetime cumulative incidence of acute anterior uveitis in a normal population and its relation to ankylosing spondylitis and histocompatibility antigen HLA-B27. Invest Ophthalmol Vis Sci 32:2568–257
20. Madden DR, Gorga JC, Strominger JL, Wiley DC (1991) The structure of HLA-B27 reveals nonamer self-peptides bound in an extended conformation. Nature 353:321–325
21. Martin TM, Zhang G, Luo J, et al. (2005) A locus on chromosome 9p predisposes to a specific disease manifestation, acute anterior uveitis, in ankylosing spondylitis, a genetically complex, multisystem, inflammatory disease. Arthritis Rheum 52:269–274
22. McCannel CA, Holland GN, Helm CJ, Cornell PJ, Winston JV, Rimmer TG (1996) Causes of uveitis in the general practice of ophthalmology. UCLA Community-Based Uveitis Study Group [comment]. Am J Ophthalmol 121:35–46
23. Medzhitov R, Janeway CA Jr (2002) Decoding the patterns of self and nonself by the innate immune system. Science 296:298–300
24. Monnet D, Breban M, Hudry C, Dougados M, Brezin AP (2004) Ophthalmic findings and frequency of extraocular manifestations in patients with HLA-B27 uveitis: a study of 175 cases. Ophthalmology 111:802–809
25. Rodriguez A, Akova YA, Pedroza-Seres M, Foster CS (1994) Posterior segment ocular manifestations in patients with HLA-B27-associated uveitis. Ophthalmology 101:1267–1274
26. Rosenbaum JT, McDevitt HO, Guss RB, Egbert PR (1980) Endotoxin-induced uveitis in rats as a model for human disease. Nature 286:611–613
27. Rothova A, van Veenedaal WG, Linssen A, Glasius E, Kijlstra A, de Jong PT (1987) Clinical features of acute anterior uveitis. Am J Ophthalmol 103:137–145
28. Rothova A, Suttorp-van Schulten MS, Frits Treffers W, Kijlstra A (1996) Causes and frequency of blindness in patients with intraocular inflammatory disease. Br J Ophthalmol 80:332–336
29. Saari KM, Paivonsalo-Hietanen T, Vaahtoranta-Lehtonen H, Tuominen J, Sillanpaa M (1995) Epidemiology of

2

endogenous uveitis in south-western Finland. Acta Ophthalmol Scand 73:345–349

30. Takeda K, Akira S (2005) Toll-like receptors in innate immunity. Int Immunol 17:1–14

31. Taurog JD, Maika SD, Simmons WA, Breban M, Hammer RE (1993) Susceptibility to inflammatory disease in HLA-B27 transgenic rat lines correlates with the level of B27 expression. J Immunol 150:4168–4178

32. Taurog JD, Richardson JA, Croft JT, et al. (1994) The germfree state prevents development of gut and joint inflammatory disease in HLA-B27 transgenic rats. J Exp Med 180:2359–2364

33. Tay-Kearney ML, Schwam BL, Lowder C, et al. (1996) Clinical features and associated systemic diseases of HLA-B27 uveitis. Am J Ophthalmol 121:47–56

34. Verma MJ, Lloyd A, Rager H, et al. (1997) Chemokines in acute anterior uveitis. Curr Eye Res 16:1202–1208

35. Wegscheider BJ, Weger M, Renner W, et al. (2005) Role of the CCL2/MCP-1 -2518A>G gene polymorphism in HLA-B27 associated uveitis. Mol Vis 11:896–900

36. Yang ZX, Liang Y, Zhu Y, et al. (2007) Increased expression of Toll-like receptor 4 in peripheral blood leucocytes and serum levels of some cytokines in patients with ankylosing spondylitis. Clin Exp Immunol 149:48–55

Chapter 3

What Can the Aqueous Humour Tell Us About Uveitis?

3

Alastair K.O. Denniston, S. John Curnow

Core Messages

- The sampling of aqueous humour (AqH) is a safe and relatively quick procedure
- Infectious agents can be identified by pathogen-specific antibody or RNA/DNA
- Non-inflamed AqH is acellular and immunosuppressive

- During episodes of uveitis, leukocytes, predominated by recently activated CD4$^+$ T cells, accumulate in the aqueous humour
- Uveitis AqH contains very high levels of locally produced pro-inflammatory cytokines and chemokines
- These pro-inflammatory molecules likely contribute to the persistence of inflammation

3.1 Clinical Examination of the Aqueous Humour in Uveitis

3.1.1 Introduction

The eye, and in particular the anterior segment, is one of the very few parts of the body where inflammation can be viewed directly, in vivo and without intervention. The clinical ophthalmologist is familiar with this privilege and uses it not only in diagnosis (i.e. to identify the site and nature of disease), but to monitor disease activity (e.g. to assess whether the inflammation is worsening or improving in response to treatment).

3.1.2 Observable Changes During Intraocular Inflammation

In most forms of uveitis there is evidence of inflammatory activity in the anterior chamber. This is primarily reflected in the cellular and non-cellular constituents of the aqueous humour (AqH), the fluid which fills the anterior chamber and bathes the inner surface of the cornea, the iris, the ciliary body and the lens. Under healthy noninflammatory conditions, the AqH is generally acellular (there are exceptions to this) and transparent. Under inflammatory conditions, there is leukocyte recruitment to the anterior segment (observed as cells in the anterior chamber) and breakdown of the blood–ocular barrier (seen as a loss of transparency of the AqH, known as

flare). Cellular activity (i.e. an indication of the number of cells present in the anterior chamber) is calculated from the number of cells seen in a 1 mm × 1 mm illuminated slit graded on a scale from 0 ($n < 1$ cells) to 4+ (>50 cells) [19]. Flare is graded from 0 (none; i.e. completely transparent) to 4+ (intense: fibrin or plastic aqueous) [19]. Flare can be more accurately measured with instruments such as the Kowa laser flare cell meter; however, this is currently used primarily in the research setting. In addition, cells circulating in the AqH may adhere to the corneal endothelium, and be visible as "keratic precipitates" on the inner aspect of the cornea. These may persist after the episode of acute inflammation, and may become pigmented over time, giving an indication of their chronicity. Certain patterns of keratic precipitates are regarded as being typical of particular forms of uveitis (for example the stellate keratic precipitates of Fuchs' heterochromic cyclitis), thus providing additional diagnostic information. Imaging of these keratic precipitates by in vivo confocal microscopy has confirmed that there are differences in the keratic precipitates seen in infectious and noninfectious uveitis, and that their morphology changes over time [40].

Where the site of inflammation is primarily the anterior uvea (anterior uveitis), the presence of cells and flare in the AqH will be the predominating feature, and will usually be accompanied by some injection of the circumlimbal vessels (seen as redness of the conjunctiva around the margin of the cornea). In intermediate uveitis, cells and flare may again be seen in the anterior chamber, but

3

are far exceeded by the degree of cells and flare in the vitreous humour, which indicates that the vitreous is the primary site of inflammation. In a true posterior uveitis, the anterior chamber will be "quiet" (i.e. no cells or flare). Commonly, however, more severe posterior segment inflammation would be accompanied by some degree of anterior involvement (seen as cells and flare in the AqH), and it is then described as a panuveitis.

3.1.3 Sampling of Aqueous Humour

It will be apparent from the above discussion that whilst clinical examination of the AqH is sufficient to diagnose the presence and severity of anterior uveal inflammation, it gives relatively limited information regarding the underlying cause of inflammation. It should be remembered that most cases of uveitis are of unknown cause, and are in fact grouped into clinical syndromes (e.g. idiopathic acute anterior uveitis, Fuchs' heterochromic cyclitis, pars planitis) on the basis of key symptoms and signs, rather than into aetiological categories. However, additional diagnostic information can be provided by the laboratory analysis of AqH, which has reaped significant benefits in both clinical and research settings.

In routine clinical care, the sampling of AqH is generally reserved for where there is concern that the underlying cause of uveitis may be infective. For example, it is common to observe mild-to-moderate anterior segment inflammation after intraocular surgery, such as after cataract extraction. In the vast majority of cases this is thought to be post-traumatic or auto-inflammatory in nature and responds to topical corticosteroid treatment. However, in occasional cases (around 0.1% of all cataract operations), anterior segment inflammation represents intraocular infection (endophthalmitis). Since endophthalmitis is an ophthalmic emergency requiring prompt treatment with appropriate antimicrobials, rapid and reliable confirmation of an infective agent from the AqH (and/or from a sample of the vitreous humour) is essential.

In the research setting, analysis of AqH in terms of cellular content (only present in inflammation) and non-cellular content (in health and in uveitis) has advanced our understanding of the immune system in the eye under resting and inflamed conditions, and has underlined some of the differences between the various forms of uveitis.

Sampling of AqH should be performed under good visualisation at the biomicroscope ("slit lamp") or under the operating microscope. A number of techniques are described in the literature [16, 20, 27, 37]; the following reflects our standard technique which has had an excellent safety record in both operating theatre and out-

patient settings [5]. Under sterile conditions and after the administration of both topical anaesthesia and 5% povidone–iodine, a 27′ needle is inserted just anterior to the temporal limbus and introduced into the anterior chamber (Fig. 3.1). The volume of AqH that can be removed typically varies between 50 µl and 150 µl. Withdrawal of fluid should be stopped if there is any significant shallowing of the anterior chamber. The ease of the procedure and the volume that can be safely removed is very highly dependent on the depth of the anterior chamber, and thus is usually easiest in myopes and most challenging in hypermetropes.

> **Summary for the Clinician**
>
> - In the normal resting eye, the aqueous humour is transparent and acellular
> - Intraocular inflammation can be observed at the slit lamp as flare and cellular infiltrate in the anterior chamber, keratic precipitates and posterior synechiae
> - Sampling of AqH may provide valuable diagnostic information and may be performed safely in the clinic or operating theatre

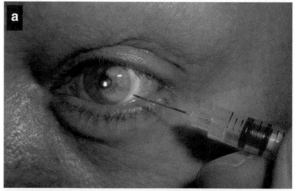

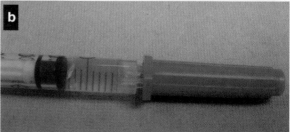

Fig. 3.1 AqH sampling in the clinical setting using a 27′ needle on a 1 ml syringe after suitable preparation with povidone–iodine and topical anaesthesia (**a**). AqH sample (approximately 150 µl) from a patient with acute anterior uveitis (**b**)

3.2 Identification of Infectious Agents in Aqueous Humour

3.2.1 Intraocular Antibody and PCR

The identification of infectious agents responsible for episodes of uveitis remains a significant problem. A number of studies have clearly demonstrated the benefit of analysing AqH for the presence of viral, bacterial and parasitic infections [11, 12]. One method is to analyse the level of intraocular antibody against a specific pathogen, which is frequently elevated in comparison to the level in the serum. In particular, determining the Goldmann–Witmer coefficient (GWC) has proved valuable. The introduction of PCR techniques increased the sensitivity of detection of the infectious agent itself in AqH (although strict control for false-positive results is required), and has allowed the development of multiplex techniques [15]. The range of infectious agents that can be detected using PCR now includes herpes simplex virus, cytomegalovirus, varicella zoster virus, *Toxoplasma gondii* and bacterial 16S rRNA. The examination of AqH by PCR for a range of infectious agents is of great value, as it is currently the only true diagnostic test available using AqH. A number of recent studies have shown the benefit of combining AqH PCR and GWC for the diagnosis of infectious uveitis, even though the majority of inflammation is contained within the posterior chamber [13, 29, 41]. An extensive analysis of suspected infectious posterior uveitis from immunocompetent and immunocompromised individuals revealed a good degree of concordance between intraocular antibody and real-time PCR [29]. There were still significant numbers that were only detectable by one of the methods, highlighting the benefit of a combined approach. The combined analysis of intraocular antibody production and PCR for viral DNA has also implicated rubella virus in the pathogenesis of Fuchs' heterochromic cyclitis (FHC) [12, 15].

3.2.2 Recent Technological Advances

Despite these two approaches, many suspected cases of infectious posterior uveitis may still require analysis of the vitreous for further investigation, and even then may remain negative. It is unclear if these reflect a failure to detect an infection, or if this indicates that they are truly idiopathic cases of posterior uveitis. Recent technological advances are leading to the development of high throughput "saturation sequencing" techniques [18] that will identify microbial organisms involved in ocular inflammation. These technologies essentially sequence all of the material present in the sample, providing a genomic representation of any organism present, and are currently being developed for the analysis of AqH (Prof. R. Van Gelder, Seattle, USA, personal communication).

> **Summary for the Clinician**
>
> - Analysis of AqH can identify specific pathogens, providing diagnostic information that will affect subsequent treatment of the disease
> - The measurement of both pathogen-specific antibodies and RNA/DNA by PCR amplification may be required for pathogen identification
> - New methods that are currently under development may allow the full sequencing of all non-human RNA/DNA in the AqH sample, allowing the identification of rare and novel pathogens

3.3 Leukocyte Populations in Aqueous Humour

3.3.1 The Noninflamed Eye

Under normal conditions, the AqH remains free of inflammatory cells, ensuring a clear visual axis. However, within the tissues there are clearly a number of resident leukocyte populations, including macrophages and dendritic cells [21]. These tissue-resident cells act as sentinel cells to respond to any inflammatory or infectious challenge that may arise.

3.3.2 Cytocentrifuge Analysis of Leukocyte Populations in Uveitis Aqueous Humour

In contrast to the situation in the noninflamed eye, the AqH can contain a very large number of leukocytes during episodes of uveitis. The most extreme example of this is the formation of a hypopyon, which is essentially a large collection of leukocytes that sediment at the bottom of the anterior chamber. A number of techniques can be used to study the inflammatory cells found in AqH. The most simple of these is to cytocentrifuge the cell suspension onto a glass slide and stain with a differential stain. When using this method, we have found that the total number of cells correlates very well with the clinical measurement of anterior chamber cells, as would be expected (Fig. 3.2a). Analysis of active uveitis AqH typically shows a mixed leukocyte infiltrate composed of lymphocytes, neutrophils and macrophages (Fig. 3.2b). However, the proportions of each population can change between

3

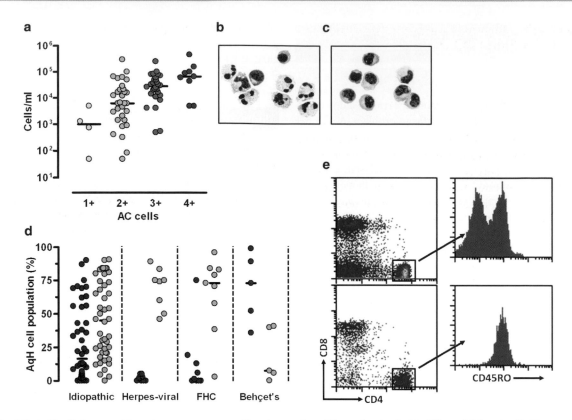

Fig. 3.2 AqH cells from uveitis patients were cytocentrifuged onto glass slides and stained with differential dyes (**a–d**). The number (**a**) and proportion (D; *red* = neutrophil, *green* = lymphocyte) of each leukocyte population were calculated. Cytocentrifuged AqH cells are shown for idiopathic uveitis (**b**) and herpes-viral uveitis (**c**). Cells were also labelled with combinations of fluorochrome-conjugated antibodies and analysed by flow cytometry (**e**). The expression of CD45RO on peripheral blood (*top panel*) and AqH (*bottom panel*) CD4+ T cells was determined by applying a gate on CD4 expression as shown. *FHC*, Fuchs' heterochromic cyclitis

different types of uveitis (Fig. 3.2c,d). The majority of idiopathic or HLA-B27, anterior or panuveitis AqH contain a predominance of lymphocytes. This distribution varies considerably, even within patients with idiopathic uveitis, which may reflect differences such as the disease aetiology or time of AqH sampling. The most extreme examples of a bias in leukocyte distribution can be found when examining herpes-viral uveitis or Fuchs' heterochromic cyclitis, where neutrophils are almost absent (Fig. 3.2d).

3.3.3 Flow Cytometric Analysis of Uveitis Aqueous Humour

Although the analysis of AqH cells by this method can reveal very useful information, other techniques, including multi-colour flow cytometry, can provide more detailed data. By labelling cells from AqH with a number of different monoclonal antibodies, each labelled with a different fluorochrome, multiple different leukocyte populations can be identified. A relatively simple analysis shows that the CD4+ lymphocyte population is composed entirely of antigen-experienced cells expressing CD45RO, as compared to the peripheral blood that contains both naive and primed cells (Fig. 3.2e). The ratio of CD4 to CD8 T cells is maintained within the AqH, although there is often a further increase in the relative frequency of CD4+ T cells as compared to peripheral blood [3]. In Behçet's disease there is a reversal of ratios, with CD8+ T cells dominating [43]. The expression of CD69 and HLA-DR on CD4+ AqH T cells suggests that they have recently been activated, in common with many other sites of inflammation [14, 39]. However, the original reports of elevated CD25 (IL-2Rα) expression [14, 25, 26] as an indicator of T cell activation now require re-evaluation, as this molecule is also expressed at high levels on regulatory T cells. AqH T cells from patients with uveitis produce IFNγ and IL-10 upon ex vivo stimulation [17], and T cell clones derived from AqH cells can secrete chemokines, including MIP1α, MIP1β and RANTES [35].

3.3.4 Antigen Specificity of Aqueous Humour T Cells

The majority of noninfectious uveitis is considered to be an autoimmune disease. However, there is little direct evidence to support this contention. Analysis of AqH T cells has suggested that antigen-specific T cells can be isolated, but this has mostly only been possible for infectious uveitis. CD4+ T cell lines generated from the AqH of patients with VZV-induced uveitis showed recognition of VZV antigen-pulsed B cells [23], and using T cell clones from these lines, the specific VZV peptide sequences recognised were identified [22]. A clear link to autoimmunity has been established for Vogt–Koyanagi–Harada disease, where ocular infiltrating T cells were found to have specificity for peptides from the melanocyte antigen tyrosinase [33]. Intriguingly, these T cells showed cross-reactive recognition of both tyrosinase and the cytomegalovirus envelope glycoprotein H, suggesting that the disease may have been initiated through a process of molecular mimicry [32]. Whether the majority of idiopathic and HLA-B27 uveitis is truly autoimmune, or merely inflammatory, remains to be determined, and will require a more extensive analysis of the specificities of AqH T cells.

3.4 Changes in the Aqueous Humour Microenvironment During Episodes of Uveitis

3.4.1 Immunological Properties of Aqueous Humour

Although the majority of studies have focused on examining the cells present in AqH, or the cytokines present in them (see below), there has also been progress in understanding how changes in the composition of AqH during episodes of uveitis might affect the functioning of the immune system. The ocular microenvironment has also been shown to modulate the expression of the chemokine receptor CXCR4. This effect was predominantly mediated by TGFβ2 in noninflammatory AqH, with less activity when AqH was from uveitis patients before starting glucocorticoid treatment [9]. Interestingly, the glucocorticoid treatment itself was able to up-regulate CXCR4 to very high levels. Early reports indicated that AqH from noninflamed eyes has the capacity to induce T cell apoptosis, and that this might therefore contribute to maintaining immune privilege [10]. However, very few AqH lymphocytes from recent-onset anterior uveitis were apoptotic [8]. AqH from uveitis patients, but not controls, were able to inhibit T cell apoptosis in vitro through IL-6 trans-signalling [8]. However, in another report, apoptosis was detected in some uveitis AqH T cells [14], suggesting that the induction of apoptosis can occur, possibly later on in the disease course, resulting in the resolution of disease.

Summary for the Clinician

- Leukocytes are normally absent from the noninflamed eye
- The frequency of neutrophils, macrophages and lymphocytes can be simply determined from cytocentrifuge preparations of AqH cells
- AqH from Fuchs' heterochromic cyclitis and herpes-viral uveitis are dominated by lymphocytes, whereas AqH from patients with Behçet's predominantly contains neutrophils
- Flow cytometry can provide a detailed profile of the different populations of lymphocytes present in AqH, and indicates that the majority of cells are recently activated CD4+ T cells
- Antigen-specific T cells have been identified in the AqH of Vogt–Koyanagi–Harada and VZV-induced uveitis

3.4.2 Cytokine Profiles of Aqueous Humour

The eye is considered to be a site of immune privilege, where immune responses are sufficiently controlled to avoid significant nonspecific pathological damage to the delicate tissues of the visual axis. A number of mechanisms have been described that maintain this privileged state [31], including the presence of a number of immunosuppressive molecules within the AqH [36]. These molecules include TGFβ2, vasoactive intestinal peptide (VIP), α-melanocyte-stimulating hormone (α-MSH), somatostatin, cortisol and calcitonin gene-related peptide (CGRP). These molecules share the ability to inhibit T cell proliferation and enhance the generation of regulatory T cell populations.

During episodes of active uveitis, the AqH microenvironment changes dramatically, from one dominated by immunosuppressive molecules to a predominance of

3

inflammatory cytokines and chemokines [7]. Initial studies of inflammatory cytokines in uveitis AqH were limited by the volume of fluid available, with ELISA methods used for analysis. Despite these limitations, a number of cytokines and chemokines have been shown to increase in the majority of patients with uveitis [7]. More recently, multiplex bead-based immunoassays have been used to simultaneously measure many different inflammatory and regulatory cytokines and chemokines [6, 28, 34, 38]. This methodology allows the simultaneous analysis of a number of different molecules in each sample, reducing the confounding factors of technical error and the large amount of disease variation in uveitis. These results revealed that the most common form of uveitis, idiopathic or HLA-B27 anterior uveitis, is characterised by an increase in the pro-inflammatory cytokines IL-1β, IL-6, IFNγ and IL-8, as well as the chemokines MCP-1 and RANTES. Concomitant with these increases was a decrease in the levels of the immunosuppressive molecule TGFβ2 [6]. Due to the large number of data points that are generated by measuring a large number of different molecules in every sample, it is necessary to perform some form of bioinformatic analysis. This can include cluster analysis (Fig. 3.3), where samples with similar profiles of cytokines and chemokines are grouped next

to each other, and similarly for the cytokines themselves. Our analysis of uveitis AqH revealed that the majority of noninflammatory samples group together, as do the AqH from idiopathic uveitis. The most interesting observations were that, despite the small sample numbers, cluster analysis grouped 2/4 herpes-viral, 4/5 FHC and 3/4 Behçet's uveitis AqH (Fig. 3.3).

Analysis of AqH from patients with Behçet's uveitis showed much greater increases in the cytokines IFNγ and TNFα [1], supporting recent evidence of the beneficial effects of anti-TNFα therapy for Behçet's disease. A similar approach analysing uveitis in childhood revealed similar elevations in IL-6 and IFNγ, although there were more frequent elevations in the T cell-derived cytokines IL-2, IL-4, IL-10 and IL-13 [30]. There were also elevations in the T cell chemoattractants RANTES and IP-10.

3.4.3   IL-10 In Aqueous Humour

Analysis of AqH from infectious uveitis also showed increases in inflammatory molecules, but in most studies there were also elevations in the regulatory cytokine IL-10 [6, 34, 38]. The significance of these findings has not been further addressed, but may be related to the

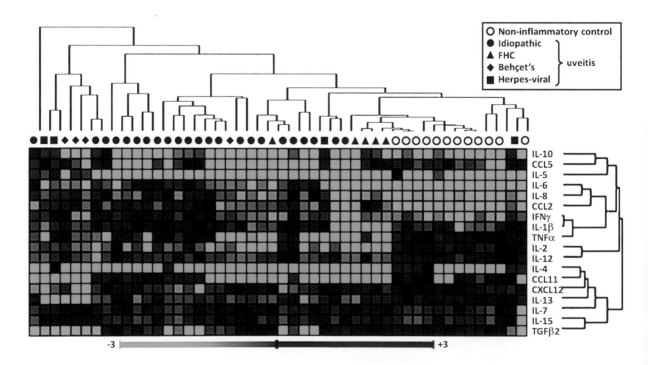

Fig. 3.3 Cluster analysis of cytokines and chemokines in non-inflammatory and uveitis AqH. The relative levels of each cytokine are represented as a colour scale, with *green* indicating no or little cytokine, and *red* a relatively high level of cytokine. Across the top of the cluster plot, the samples are grouped next to those with the closest profile of all of the molecules tested. Also, on the right hand side is a similar association for the cytokines and chemokines. *FHC*, Fuchs' heterochromic cyclitis. Figure adapted from [9]

induction of regulatory T cell populations that secrete high levels of IL-10 [24]. It is important to note that the presence of IL-10 has also been used to suggest a diagnosis of primary intraocular lymphoma. A recent study concluded that a 30 pg ml^{-1} cut-off of IL-10 in AqH provides a sensitivity of 0.96, but a specificity of only 0.84 [4]. A number of studies have suggested that by measuring the levels of both IL-6 and IL-10 it may be possible to distinguish lymphoma [2, 42], as IL-6 is present at only very low levels in lymphoma. However, the analysis of larger numbers of samples for both IL-10 and IL-6 will be required to provide accurate sensitivity and specificity values for this potentially useful diagnostic tool.

Summary for the Clinician

- Under noninflammatory conditions AqH is an immunosuppressive microenvironment, containing TGFβ2, α-MSH, VIP and CGRP
- During episodes of uveitis, many inflammatory cytokines and chemokines increase to high levels in AqH
- The inflamed AqH microenvironment likely contributes to the persistence of inflammation through activation of the endothelium, recruitment of more leukocytes, and maintenance of the infiltrate through the inhibition of apoptosis

3.5 Summary and Future Directions

Examination of AqH has taught us much about the normal state of the eye, and more particularly how it is modified during episodes of uveitis. The clinician has always benefitted from the ability to observe disease activity without resorting to invasive techniques. By sampling AqH, a relatively safe and noninvasive procedure, and employing cutting-edge laboratory techniques, it is now possible to gain much more information on the disease aetiology, pathogenesis and potential for treatment. This information allows us to better define the aetiology and pathology of uveitis, and in the future should provide better prognostic information and identify new therapeutic targets.

References

1. Ahn JK, Yu HG, Chung H, Park YG (2006) Intraocular cytokine environment in active Behcet uveitis. Am J Ophthalmol 142:429–434

2. Buggage RR, Whitcup SM, Nussenblatt RB, Chan CC (1999) Using interleukin 10 to interleukin 6 ratio to distinguish primary intraocular lymphoma and uveitis. Invest Ophthalmol Vis Sci 40:2462–2463

3. Calder VL, Shaer B, Muhaya M, Mclauchlan M, Pearson RV, Jolly G, Towler HM, Lightman S (1999) Increased CD4+ expression and decreased IL-10 in the anterior chamber in idiopathic uveitis. Invest Ophthalmol Vis Sci 40:2019–2024

4. Cassoux N, Giron A, Bodaghi B, Tran TH, Baudet S, Davy F, Chan CC, Lehoang P, Merle-Beral H (2007) IL-10 measurement in aqueous humor for screening patients with suspicion of primary intraocular lymphoma. Invest Ophthalmol Vis Sci 48:3253–3259

5. Cheung CM, Durrani OM, Murray PI (2004) The safety of anterior chamber paracentesis in patients with uveitis. Br J Ophthalmol 88:582–583

6. Curnow SJ, Murray PI (2006) Inflammatory mediators of uveitis: cytokines and chemokines. Curr Opin Ophthalmol 17:532–537

7. Curnow SJ, Scheel-Toellner D, Jenkinson W, Raza K, Durrani OM, Faint JM, Rauz S, Wloka K, Pilling D, Rose-John S, Buckley CD, Murray PI, Salmon M (2004) Inhibition of T cell apoptosis in the aqueous humor of patients with uveitis by IL-6/soluble IL-6 receptor trans-signaling. J Immunol 173:5290–5297

8. Curnow SJ, Wloka K, Faint JM, Amft N, Cheung CM, Savant V, Lord J, Akbar AN, Buckley CD, Murray PI, Salmon M(2004) Topical glucocorticoid therapy directly induces up-regulation of functional CXCR4 on primed T lymphocytes in the aqueous humor of patients with uveitis. J Immunol 172:7154–7161

9. Curnow SJ, Falciani F, Durrani OM, Cheung CM, Ross EJ, Wloka K, Rauz S, Wallace GR, Salmon M, Murray PI (2005) Multiplex bead immunoassay analysis of aqueous humor reveals distinct cytokine profiles in uveitis. Invest Ophthalmol Vis Sci 46:4251–4259

10. D'Orazio TJ, DeMarco BM, Mayhew ES, Niederkorn JY (1999) Effect of aqueous humor on apoptosis of inflammatory cell types. Invest Ophthalmol Vis Sci 40:1418–1426

11. de Boer JH, Verhagen C, Bruinenberg M, Rothova A, de Jong PT, Baarsma GS, Van der LA, Ooyman FM, Bollemeijer JG, Derhaag PJ, Kijlstra A (1996) Serologic and polymerase chain reaction analysis of intraocular fluids in the diagnosis of infectious uveitis. Am J Ophthalmol 121:650–658

12. de Groot-Mijnes JD, de VL, Rothova A, Schuller M, van Loon AM, Weersink AJ (2006) Rubella virus is associated with Fuchs heterochromic iridocyclitis. Am J Ophthalmol 141:212–214

13. de Groot-Mijnes JD, Rothova A, van Loon AM, Schuller M, Ten Dam-van Loon NH, de Boer JH, Schuurman R, Weersink AJ (2006) Polymerase chain reaction and Goldmann-Witmer coefficient analysis are complimentary

for the diagnosis of infectious uveitis. Am J Ophthalmol 141:313–318

14. Dick AD, Siepmann K, Dees C, Duncan L, Broderick C, Liversidge J, Forrester JV (1999) Fas-Fas ligand-mediated apoptosis within aqueous during idiopathic acute anterior uveitis. Invest Ophthalmol Vis Sci 40:2258–2267

15. Dworkin LL, Gibler TM, Van Gelder RN (2002) Real-time quantitative polymerase chain reaction diagnosis of infectious posterior uveitis. Arch Ophthalmol 120:1534–1539

16. Grewal SP (1989) A technique for paracentesis. Ophthalmic Surg 20:525

17. Hill T, Galatowicz G, Akerele T, Lau CH, Calder V, Lightman S (2005) Intracellular T lymphocyte cytokine profiles in the aqueous humour of patients with uveitis and correlation with clinical phenotype. Clin Exp Immunol 139:132–137

18. Hillier LW, Marth GT, Quinlan AR, Dooling D, Fewell G, Barnett D, Fox P, Glasscock JI, Hickenbotham M, Huang W, Magrini VJ, Richt RJ, Sander SN, Stewart DA, Stromberg M, Tsung EF, Wylie T, Schedl T, Wilson RK, Mardis ER (2008) Whole-genome sequencing and variant discovery in *C. elegans*. Nat Methods 5:183–188

19. Jabs DA, Nussenblatt RB, Rosenbaum JT (2005) Standardization of uveitis nomenclature for reporting clinical data. Results of the First International Workshop. Am J Ophthalmol 140:509–516

20. May DR, Noll FG (1988) An improved approach to aqueous paracentesis. Ophthalmic Surg 19:821–822

21. McMenamin PG (1997) The distribution of immune cells in the uveal tract of the normal eye. Eye 11(Pt 2):183–193

22. Milikan JC, Kuijpers RW, Baarsma GS, Osterhaus AD, Verjans GM (2006) Characterization of the varicella zoster virus (VZV)-specific intra-ocular T-cell response in patients with VZV-induced uveitis. Exp Eye Res 83:69–75

23. Milikan JC, Kinchington PR, Baarsma GS, Kuijpers RW, Osterhaus AD, Verjans GM (2007) Identification of viral antigens recognized by ocular infiltrating T cells from patients with varicella zoster virus-induced uveitis. Invest Ophthalmol Vis Sci 48:3689–3697

24. Mills KH, McGuirk P (2004) Antigen-specific regulatory T cells—their induction and role in infection. Semin Immunol 16:107–117

25. Muhaya M, Calder V, Towler HM, Shaer B, Mclauchlan M, Lightman S (1998) Characterization of T cells and cytokines in the aqueous humour (AH) in patients with Fuchs' heterochromic cyclitis (FHC) and idiopathic anterior uveitis (IAU). Clin Exp Immunol 111:123–128

26. Muhaya M, Calder VL, Towler HM, Jolly G, Mclauchlan M, Lightman S (1999) Characterization of phenotype and cytokine profiles of T cell lines derived from vitreous humour in ocular inflammation in man. Clin Exp Immunol 116:410–414

27. O'Rourke J, Taylor DM, McDonald P, Kreutzer DL (1991) An aqueous paracentesis pipet. Ophthalmic Surg 22:166–167

28. Ooi KG, Galatowicz G, Towler HM, Lightman SL, Calder VL (2006) Multiplex cytokine detection versus ELISA for aqueous humor: IL-5, IL-10, and IFNγ profiles in uveitis. Invest Ophthalmol Vis Sci 47:272–277

29. Rothova A, de Boer JH, Ten Dam-van Loon NH, Postma G, de VL, Zuurveen SJ, Schuller M, Weersink AJ, van Loon AM, de Groot-Mijnes JD (2008) Usefulness of aqueous humor analysis for the diagnosis of posterior uveitis. Ophthalmology 115:306–311

30. Sijssens KM, Rijkers GT, Rothova A, Stilma JS, Schellekens PA, de Boer JH (2007) Cytokines, chemokines and soluble adhesion molecules in aqueous humor of children with uveitis. Exp Eye Res 85:443–449

31. Streilein JW (2003) Ocular immune privilege: the eye takes a dim but practical view of immunity and inflammation. J Leukoc Biol 74:179–185

32. Sugita S, Takase H, Taguchi C, Imai Y, Kamoi K, Kawaguchi T, Sugamoto Y, Futagami Y, Itoh K, Mochizuki M (2006) Ocular infiltrating CD4+ T cells from patients with Vogt–Koyanagi–Harada disease recognize human melanocyte antigens. Invest Ophthalmol Vis Sci 47:2547–2554

33. Sugita S, Takase H, Kawaguchi T, Taguchi C, Mochizuki M (2007) Cross-reaction between tyrosinase peptides and cytomegalovirus antigen by T cells from patients with Vogt–Koyanagi–Harada disease. Int Ophthalmol 27:87–95

34. Takase H, Futagami Y, Yoshida T, Kamoi K, Sugita S, Imai Y, Mochizuki M (2006) Cytokine profile in aqueous humor and sera of patients with infectious or noninfectious uveitis. Invest Ophthalmol Vis Sci 47:1557–1561

35. Takase H, Sugita S, Taguchi C, Imai Y, Mochizuki M (2006) Capacity of ocular infiltrating T helper type 1 cells of patients with non-infectious uveitis to produce chemokines. Br J Ophthalmol 90:765–768

36. Taylor A (2003) A review of the influence of aqueous humor on immunity. Ocul Immunol Inflamm 11:231–241

37. Van der LA, Rothova A (1997) Diagnostic anterior chamber paracentesis in uveitis: a safe procedure? Br J Ophthalmol 81:976–979

38. van KB, Rothova A, Rijkers GT, de Groot-Mijnes JD (2006) Distinct cytokine and chemokine profiles in the aqueous of patients with uveitis and cystoid macular edema. Am J Ophthalmol 142:192–194

39. Wang XC, Norose K, Yano A, Ohta K, Segawa K (1995) Two-color flow cytometric analysis of activated T lymphocytes in aqueous humor of patients with endogenous vs. exogenous uveitis. Curr Eye Res 14:425–433

40. Wertheim MS, Mathers WD, Planck SJ, Martin TM, Suhler EB, Smith JR, Rosenbaum JT (2004) In vivo confocal microscopy of keratic precipitates. Arch Ophthalmol 122:1773–1781

41. Westeneng, C, Rothova A, de Boer JH, de Groot-Mijnes JD (2007) Infectious uveitis in immunocompromised patients and the diagnostic value of polymerase chain reaction and Goldmann–Witmer coefficient in aqueous analysis. Am J Ophthalmol 144:781–785

42. Whitcup SM, Stark-Vancs V, Wittes RE, Solomon D, Podgor MJ, Nussenblatt RB, Chan CC (1997) Association of interleukin 10 in the vitreous and cerebrospinal fluid and primary central nervous system lymphoma. Arch Ophthalmol 115:1157–1160

43. Yu HG, Lee DS, Seo JM, Ahn JK, Yu YS, Lee WJ, Chung H (2004) The number of CD8+ T cells and NKT cells increases in the aqueous humor of patients with Behcet's uveitis. Clin Exp Immunol 137:437–443

Is Diabetic Retinopathy an Inflammatory Disease? Inflammation as a Stimulus for Vascular Leakage and Proliferation

4

Antonia M. Joussen

Core Messages

- Diabetic retinopathy shows many of the characteristics of an inflammatory disease. Diabetic retinal neovascularization, as well as vascular leakage, capillary nonperfusion and endothelial cell damage, are caused, in part, by retinal leukostasis.
- In diabetes, leukocytes adhere to the retinal vasculature via intercellular adhesion molecule-1 (ICAM-1) and CD18. FasL-mediated apoptosis is involved in vascular remodeling upon ischemia and diabetes.
- Macular edema is the major cause of blindness in diabetics, and results from either inflammation, metabolic alterations, ischemia, hydrostatic and mechanical forces or a combination thereof.
- Blood–retinal barrier breakdown may occur to a variable extent via three possible mechanisms: dysfunction of the intercellular junctions, increased transcellular transport, or increased endothelial cell destruction.
- In early experimental diabetes, vascular endothelial growth factor (VEGF) plays key roles in mediating both ischemia-related neovascularization as well as retinal leukostasis. These pathological processes are similar to those underlying the leukocyte-mediated pruning of the retinal vasculature during normal development.
- Phase II studies with VEGF inhibitors have shown their effect on diabetic macula edema for clinically relevant endpoints. Further studies are warranted to determine their superiority over steroid-based therapies (e.g., triamcinolone) in terms of effectiveness at reducing macula edema.

4.1 Introduction

4.1.1 Clinical Problems and Cellular Interaction in Diabetic Retinopathy

Diabetic macular edema is the most common cause of visual impairment in patients with diabetes mellitus, and it affects approximately 75,000 new patients in the United States every year [14, 65, 66]. The incidence of macular edema significantly increases with increasing severity of diabetes in both early-onset and late-onset diabetic patients [65, 66].

Diabetic macular edema tends to be a chronic disease. Although spontaneous recovery is not uncommon, 24% of eyes with clinically significant macular edema (CSME) and 33% of eyes with center-involving CSME will have a moderate visual loss (15 or more letters on the ETDRS chart) within three years if untreated [27, 31].

An increase in passive permeability through the endothelium can occur via three general mechanisms:
- Dysfunction of the intercellular junctions
- Increased transcellular transport
- Increased endothelial cell destruction

The initial site of damage that results in the increased vascular permeability is controversial to date. Although the impairment of perivascular supporting cells such as pericytes and glial cells might play a role, endothelial cell dysfunction and injury seem more likely to be the first pathogenetic step towards the breakdown of the blood–retinal barrier early in the course of the disease. The pathogenesis of this is tightly related to a low-grade inflammation leading to an increased leukocyte-adhesion to the vascular endothelium and infiltration of the retinal tissue.

The second major problem in diabetic retinopathy is proliferation, leading to hemorrhage and ultimately to fibrovascular proliferation and associated tractional retinal detachment, causing visual loss.

In the past few decades, our knowledge of the mechanisms underlying retinal vasoproliferation has increased greatly. While vasoproliferation was once considered to be mainly a consequence of ischemia, current evidence also supports a contribution from inflammatory mechanisms. Inflammation is also highly related to vascular leakage in diseases that are known to result in retinal and macular edema. Recently, inflammatory mechanisms have gained interest in relation to retinal pathology following ischemia, as well as diseases such as diabetic retinopathy (DR) and sickle cell retinopathy.

The definition of inflammation in this setting is the involvement of any leukocyte-mediated pathology in the course of the disease. We will discuss several lines of evidence, including correlative studies of elevated levels of inflammatory mediators in the presence of DR and the impact of anti-inflammatory agents on the disease. As a central focus in the second section, we will discuss a series of preclinical studies that support a causal linkage between inflammation and two principal characteristics of the pathology associated with DR, ischemia-linked neovascularization and the breakdown of the blood–retinal barrier (BRB), together with the role of VEGF in mediating these events.

4.1.2 Elevated Adhesion Molecules and Inflammatory Mediators in Diabetic Retinopathy

Both clinical and preclinical studies have associated the development of DR with elevated ocular levels of inflammatory mediators. McLeod et al. [75] reported that levels of intercellular adhesion molecule-1 (ICAM-1), an important adhesive molecule for circulating leukocytes, were elevated throughout the vasculature of diabetic patients, whereas the distribution was much more restricted in nondiabetic subjects; moreover, this elevation was accompanied by a significantly higher number of neutrophils in both the choroid and retina. Limb et al. [72] reported that levels of ICAM-1 as well as other adhesion molecules such as vascular cell adhesion molecule (VCAM-1) and E-selectin were elevated in patients with proliferative DR, while Funatsu [36] has also reported elevated levels of ICAM-1 in patients with diabetic macular edema (DME). These patients also showed elevated vitreous levels of VEGF [37], which upregulates ICAM-1 expression [105].

VEGF may in fact be a key factor mediating inflammatory events in the diabetic eye, and DR-correlated elevation of VEGF levels was first reported over a decade ago [1, 3]. Since then, diabetes-associated elevations of VEGF in the vitreous have been reported by a number of groups, together with increases in a variety of other factors, including interleukin-6 [35], angiotensin II [36], angiopoietin 2 [107], erythropoietin [108] and stroma-derived factor-1 (SDF-1). SDF-1 is itself a stimulator of VEGF expression [15] and an important mediator of cell migration and adhesion [67]

Tumor necrosis factor-α (TNF-α) is a proinflammatory cytokine that has also been implicated in the pathogenesis of DR [70, 71, 94]; moreover, susceptibility to DR has been associated with TNF-α gene polymorphism [44]. TNF-α is found in the extracellular matrix, endothelium, and vessel walls of fibrovascular tissue in proliferative DR [70], and in the vitreous from eyes with this complication [33, 101]. TNF-α can stimulate VEGF expression by the retinal pigment epithelium [85] and in choroidal neovascular membranes [43], and has been implicated as an inducer of pathological angiogenesis in the retina [38]. The evidence provided by these correlative measurements of inflammatory mediators has been supplemented by other approaches. The advent of high-density microarray technology [16, 24, 48, 99], with its capacity for the simultaneous monitoring of thousands of genes, provides a unique opportunity for high-throughput analysis of DR at the molecular level. In an analysis of retinal gene expression in streptozotocin-induced diabetes in rats, numerous genes operative in inflammatory reactions were found to be upregulated [55]. Prominent among these were the genes for macrophage migration inhibitory factor (MIF), a proinflammatory lymphokine that is believed to be involved in maintaining neutrophils in the vasculature and in facilitating their adhesion and local release of cytokines [84, 95], as well as a number of genes for adhesion molecules and apoptosis. While the findings from these approaches are purely correlative, and are not able to differentiate between potential molecular mechanisms, they can nonetheless provide important clues to the nature of processes that may be involved in the pathogenesis of DR. Finally, correlative studies have also been carried out by examining the levels of serum factors in patients with DR [76]. These workers reported that the levels of the chemokines RANTES (Regulated on Activation, Normal T-cell Expressed and Secreted) and SDF-1α were significantly elevated in patients with at least severe nonproliferative DR compared to patients with less severe DR. Positive immunostaining was observed in the inner retina for RANTES and monocyte chemoattractant protein-1 (MCP-1) in patients with diabetes. In keeping with earlier findings, staining was also strongly positive throughout the diabetic retina for ICAM-1, while normal retinal tissues showed little reactivity.

4.2 Inflammatory Processes Mediate Diabetic Macula Edema

4.2.1 Diabetic Vascular Leakage is Mediated by Inflammation

A series of investigations into the mechanisms underlying vascular damage in diabetes have suggested that an inflammatory process, similar to that which mediates vascular pruning, contributes to the breakdown of the BRB, with both VEGF and inflammatory leukocytes again exerting important influences.

In the specific case of DR, intravitreal injection of VEGF in monkeys led to many of the features characteristic of the diabetic pathology, including intraretinal and pre-retinal neovascularization, with the induced blood vessels characterized by endothelial cell hyperplasia, microaneurysm formation, hemorrhage and edema, capillary occlusion and ischemia [103]. Several mechanisms are believed to mediate VEGF's actions in promoting vascular leakage, including increases in endothelial cell fenestrations [90] and damage to tight junctions [8]. Of particular interest in the context of inflammatory mechanisms is VEGF's upregulation of the expression of ICAM-1. Miyamoto et al. [78], using a rodent model of diabetes, reported that the early stages of the disease were characterized by leukocyte entrapment in capillaries, followed by local nonperfusion and leakage. This leukostasis was correlated with increased expression of ICAM-1. Blockade of this ICAM-1 with a monoclonal antibody led to significant reductions in both nonperfusion and leakage [78], with concomitant reductions in diabetes-associated leukostasis and injury or death of endothelial cells [56]. Similar elevations of ICAM-1 and leukocyte numbers have also been observed in human eyes of patients with DR [75], suggesting that the animal models do reflect the human disease in this regard. These phenomena, together with increases in vascular permeability and breakdown of the blood–retinal barrier, were found to be directly correlated with increases in retinal levels of VEGF in diabetic animals [89]; in addition, these effects were blocked by suppressing VEGF action through the administration of a soluble VEGF receptor construct [61]. In a parallel experiment, intravitreally injected VEGF led to increased retinal expression of ICAM-1, together with increased leukocyte adhesion and increased vascular permeability; all of these responses were significantly reduced by intravenous administration of an antibody to ICAM-1 [78]. Finally, diabetic mice in which ICAM-1 or its leukocyte-bearing ligand CD18 have been genetically ablated show significant reductions in leukostasis and endothelial cell injury, with reductions in the number of pericyte ghosts and acellular capillaries

after 11 months [60]. Taken together, these experiments support a mechanism whereby the diabetes-associated elevation of VEGF leads to increased ICAM-1 expression, followed by increased leukocyte adhesion, endothelial cell injury and increased vascular permeability. As in the case of physiological vascular pruning, Fas/FasL-mediated apoptosis appears to be the final step in the inflammatory damage. Joussen et al. [57] reported that in streptozotocin-induced diabetes in rats, FasL expression was increased in neutrophils, while Fas expression was simultaneously upregulated in the retinal vasculature. In vitro assays revealed that leukocytes from the diabetic rats, but not from controls, could induce endothelial cell apoptosis; moreover, inhibition of FasL-mediated apoptosis in vivo by systemic administration of an anti-FasL antibody significantly inhibited endothelial cell apoptosis and BRB breakdown. Finally, these phenomena further emphasize the specifically inflammatory nature of the VEGF165 isoform. In nondiabetic rats, injection of VEGF164 (the rodent equivalent of human VEGF165) was approximately twice as potent as the rodent VEGF120 isoform in mediating upregulation of ICAM-1, leukocyte adhesion and the induction of BRB breakdown that is characteristic of diabetes [46]. These findings were accompanied by experiments in diabetic rats where intravitreous injection of pegaptanib, which specifically targets VEGF165/164, significantly inhibited leukostasis and BRB breakdown, both in early and in late diabetes [46]. Moreover, this work has proved to have direct clinical application, as intravitreous pegaptanib was found to provide significant clinical benefit in treating both the leakage characteristic of DME [23] as well as retinal revascularization in diabetic eyes [2].

4.2.2 Diabetic Vascular Leakage Can Be Inhibited by Anti-inflammatory Agents

Induction of adhesion molecules on endothelial cells by proinflammatory cytokines such as TNF-α [72] and VEGF is mediated at the molecular level by the activation of a redox-sensitive transcription factor, nuclear factor NF-κB [106]. NF-κB upregulates ICAM-1 and various inflammatory genes such as cyclooxygenase (COX)-2 [69]. The cyclooxygenases COX-1 and COX-2 are key enzymes in the conversion of arachidonic acid to prostaglandin H2, the common precursor for all other eicosanoids. COX-1 is expressed ubiquitously and generates eicosanoids with cytoprotective function, whereas COX-2 is an immediate early gene expressed at sites of acute inflammation which generates eicosanoids with a proinflammatory role that create a positive feedback loop by further activating NF-κB and inflammatory cytokines [74, 86].

The observation that arthritic diabetic patients receiving high daily doses of aspirin exhibit reduced symptoms of DR led to the hypothesis that anti-inflammatory treatment could prove beneficial [88]. Aspirin, in low doses (8 mg per day), inhibits platelet aggregation, predominantly via acetylation of COX-1 and reduction of thromboxane A2 production. In intermediate doses (2–4 g per day), aspirin inhibits both COX-1 and COX-2, blocking prostaglandin production, and is antipyretic [87]. In high doses (6–8 g per day), it is a potent anti-inflammatory drug suitable for the treatment of rheumatic disorders. The mechanism of this action is unclear, although it seems to be COX and prostaglandin-independent [109]. It should be noted, however, that while aspirin was originally found to inhibit platelet aggregation in vitro and to retard the development of microaneurysms in patients with DR [64], the results of the Early Treatment of Diabetic Retinopathy Study (ETDRS) and the Wisconsin Epidemiologic Study of Diabetic Retinopathy did not identify any beneficial effect of low and intermediate amounts of aspirin use in DR [28].

Recently, interest has arisen in the use of specific COX-2 inhibitors that do not bear the unwanted gastrointestinal side effects of general anti-inflammatory drugs such as aspirin. In a rat model of DR, aspirin and the selective COX-2 inhibitor meloxicam reduce leukostasis and vascular leakage, in part through the inhibition of TNF-α and NF-κB activation; similar results were seen with the anti-TNF-α agent etanercept, a soluble TNF-α receptor/Fc fusion protein [58]. All three agents prevented the upregulation of ICAM-1 and eNOS that is observed early in the course of DR [58]. Finally, in a clinical study, Sfikakis et al. [97] reported that intravenous administration of infliximab, a monoclonal antibody to TNF-α, led to an alleviating reduction in macular thickness, as well as an alleviation of symptoms in patients with DME. Taken together, these various findings suggest that inhibition of inflammation holds promise as a method for alleviating the retinal vascular symptoms that accompany diabetes, and simultaneously provides support for the idea that inflammation is a contributing factor to the overall retinal pathology.

4.3 Inflammatory Aspects of Retinal Vascular Remodeling and Growth

Even though there is no animal model system that accurately reproduces the entire course of clinical diabetic retinopathy, rodent models do exist which resemble the clinical condition in several respects, including the importance of retinal leukostasis. These models have demonstrated that some of the processes that contribute to vascular damage in ischemic retinal conditions are very similar to those that underlie the physiological remodeling of the nascent vasculature during normal retinal development.

- Leukocytes mediate retinal vascular remodeling during development and vaso-obliteration in disease
- VEGF and leukocyte invasion are important factors in regulating both ischemia-mediated ocular neovascularization and vascular damage in DR
- T-lymphocytes are negative regulators of pathological retinal neovascularization
- Monocytes are positive regulators of pathological retinal neovascularization
- Retinal cell injury and death are Fas/FasL-dependent

4.3.1 Leukocytes Mediate Retinal Vascular Remodeling During Development and Vaso-Obliteration in Disease

In studies of vascularization in the rat retina, Ishida et al. [45] have shown that pruning of the vasculature occurs in normal development and that similar processes are involved in the pathological obliteration of retinal vasculature during conditions of hyperoxia. During normal development, the retinal vasculature extends to fill the peripheral avascular retina; beginning on postnatal (P) day 5, these investigators reported a considerable increase in the number of adherent cells, which they identified as leukocytes using immunochemical staining for CD45 (leukocyte common antigen). The number of leukocytes subsequently decreased, reaching a plateau from P6 to P11 as the vascular pruning moved peripherally. As the vasculature grew toward the periphery, the zone containing the leukocytes also migrated toward the periphery, staying 2–3 disk diameters behind the leading edge of vascular growth. In its wake was a pruned and remodeled secondary vasculature. When the leukocyte and vascular changes were compared within a zone five disc diameters from the disc, it was apparent that the decrease in both vascular density and branch-surrounded spaces was preceded by an increase in leukocyte density, indicating a cause–effect relationship. By P12, all pruning was completed and the leukocytes had all disappeared [45]. Studies of the mechanism of local adhesion of these leukocytes revealed key roles for leukocyte integrin CD18 and its corresponding ligand, ICAM-1 [45]. Western blotting showed that ICAM-1 expression was elevated in P4–P6 retinas actively undergoing remodeling as compared to normal adult rat retinas, in which vascular remodeling was absent. Moreover, immunochemical studies in P8 retinas demonstrated that the upregulation of ICAM-1 expression was localized to the region of the vasculature containing the adherent leukocytes. In addition, there was very little ICAM-1 expression at P1 or P12, times at which there were very few leukocytes present. During the P4P6 period, when the biggest changes in leukocyte numbers and vascular density took place, CD18 inhibition by a neutralizing antibody confirmed the causal involvement of leukocytes in vascular pruning. Both the number of adherent leukocytes and the spaces in the vasculature were significantly reduced. Similarly, genetically transformed mice lacking CD18 showed much less vascular pruning at P9 than wild-type mice. Additional immunocytochemical experiments [45], using an antibody to CD8 and CD25, revealed that many of the adherent leukocytes were T-lymphocytes; moreover, administration of a neutralizing antibody to CD2, an antigen that is essential for T-lymphocyte adhesion, significantly suppressed vascular pruning [45], T-lymphocytes are the principal locus of expression of Fas, while its ligand FasL is much more widely expressed [81]. Apoptosis, mediated through the interaction of Fas–FasL, was the principal means of effecting vascular pruning; intraperitoneal administration of a FasL-neutralizing antibody led to a 75% decrease in vascular pruning at P6 [45]. These basic molecular mechanisms underlying vascular pruning during normal development were also found to be operative in a pathological model of hyperoxia-induced ischemia [45]. P2 mice, together with their nursing mothers, were placed in an 80% oxygen environment for up to 12 h, leading to dramatic vaso-obliteration. This decrease in vascularization occurred shortly after an increase in the number of adherent leukocytes. As had occurred during physiological pruning, ICAM-1 expression was elevated in parallel with leukocyte accumulation, and vaso-obliteration was significantly diminished by administration of an antibody to CD18, the ligand for ICAM-1. Similarly, CD18-deficient mice showed much less vaso-obliteration of retinal vasculature than did wild-type controls when similarly exposed to oxygen. The importance of FasL-mediated apoptosis was also confirmed, as vaso-obliteration was significantly reduced in response to administration of a FasL-neutralizing antibody [45].

The pathophysiology of DR is complex, with vascular changes including both neovascularization and damage to the existing retinal vasculature. A number of biochemical pathways are believed to be important in linking hyperglycemia to vascular abnormalities in the retina [17, 32]. Avascular capillaries and microaneurysms in the retinal vasculature, characteristic histopathologic alterations in DR, have been demonstrated in a variety of long-term animal models of diabetes [13, 25, 62, 63]. Alterations in the retinal vasculature include death of pericytes, thickening of the basement membrane, and adhesion of leukocytes to the endothelium, leading to blockages and capillary dropout, with resultant local ischemia [17, 57, 77]. These phenomena reflect an accelerated death rate in both pericytes and endothelial cells, which is evident before the capillary dropouts [79].

4.3.2 Effects of VEGF on Ocular Neovascularisation and Vascular Permeability

VEGF is a pluripotent growth factor which exhibits a number of properties that are important in promoting both the ischemia-promoted neovascularization and the vascular leakage that are characteristic of DR. It is the most potent known promoter of angiogenesis, acting in a variety of roles, including endothelial cell mitogen, chemoattractant and survival factor ([5, 9, 68]; see [30] for a review), and an extensive body of research has established its importance for ocular vascularizing diseases (reviewed in [82]). It should be noted, moreover, that VEGF is upregulated by hypoxia [30], a direct consequence of the local nonperfusion and ischemia [20]. Retinal cell types that express VEGF and which respond to hypoxia by its upregulation include all classes of neurons, glia, endothelial cells, pericytes, and the retinal pigment epithelium [4, 12, 29]. As discussed above, VEGF is a key mediator of ocular neovascularization; the following sections discuss recent studies in rodent model systems that have provided further clues as to the mechanisms that mediate its actions in promoting both neovascularization in DR and the breakdown of the BRB.

Ishida et al. [47] have provided evidence that VEGF plays a key role in ischemia-mediated retinal vascularization, and that this process is both positively and negatively regulated by inflammatory cells. Using a mouse model system approximating retinopathy of prematurity, they induced the formation of an ischemic retina through exposure to a high oxygen environment; when oxygen levels were returned to normal, an aberrant neovascularization ensued, with proliferation into the vitreous. This pathological revascularization was compared to the physiological vascularization that occurs during retinal development [47]. During physiological vascularization, retinal VEGF levels were upregulated, with the VEGF164 isoform approximately twice as abundant as VEGF120. VEGF levels were further increased during pathological vascularization, with most of the increase occurring with VEGF164, which reached levels more than tenfold greater than VEGF120. The importance of VEGF for both forms of vascularization was demonstrated by their inhibition following intravitreous injection of a VEGF receptor–FC fusion protein, which inactivates all VEGF isoforms. Interestingly, injection of pegaptanib, an aptamer which binds VEGF164 but not VEGF120, was just as effective as the fusion protein in inhibiting pathological vascularization, while having little effect on physiological vascularization [47].

The inflammatory nature of the ischemia-induced pathological vascularization was further evidenced by the accumulation of adherent leukocytes on the leading edge of the pathological vascularization very shortly after induction of growth; these leukocytes were not present at very early stages of physiologic vascularization. Moreover, as had been seen during both physiologic and pathologic vascular pruning (see above), immunohistochemical studies revealed the presence of T-lymphocytes on the pathologic vascular fronds. Inactivation of T-lymphocytes with a neutralizing antibody to CD2 led to a significant increase in pathologic vascularization, suggesting that they were acting to control its extent [47].

Finally, an additional feature of the pathologic vascularization was the presence of monocytes, identified immunohistochemically. Inactivation of monocytes by clodronate liposomes significantly reduced the pathological vascularization, but not physiological vascularization [47]. Similar findings have been reported by several other groups [26, 96, 104]. As circulating monocytes are both attracted by VEGF [11, 19, 105] and also express it [41], especially in conditions of hypoxia [47], this component of the inflammatory response may serve as an amplificatory mechanism, while T-lymphocyte-mediated apoptosis serves as a negative control.

4.4 Clinical Application of the Inflammatory Concept in Diabetic Retinopathy

Anti-inflammatory treatment has reached clinical application. Even though still considered an "off-label" use, triamcinolone has been effectively used for macular edema, and comparative studies are required to determine its effect in relation to anti-VEGF medication.

4.4.1 Nonsteroidal Anti-inflammatory Drugs

As cyclooxygenase inhibitors (NSAIDs) block the synthesis and release of prostaglandins, nonsteroidal drugs have been investigated in the prophylaxis and therapy of postsurgical cystoid macular edema. It is clear that NSAIDs target the inflammatory mediators that are responsible for the edema formation, and although they may not be an optimal standalone treatment, they can be used as steroid-sparing agents. There may be several

reasons why NSAIDs cannot improve vision in diabetic macular edema, such as chronic edema, inflammation and ischemia that induce permanent structural alterations. Although effects on diabetic vascular leakage were achieved in preclinical studies [58, 59], there is so far no clinical evidence for an effect of NSAIDs in diabetic macular edema.

4.4.2 Corticosteroids

Steroids are currently regaining attention with the growing use of intravitreal triamcinolone. Corticosteroids block the release of arachidonic acid from cell membranes and thus reduce the synthesis of prostaglandins. Furthermore, they inhibit the migration of leukocytes and the release of proinflammatory mediators such as TNF-α and VEGF. Steroids specifically stabilize endothelial tight junctions and increase their numbers [7, 92]. As discussed previously, this is especially important to the development of macular edema. Routes of administration are manifold, including topical, periocular, oral, and intravenous routes. Subtenon injections of corticosteroids are widely used in patients with asymmetric or unilateral uveitis [111]. The advantages of the periocular injections are high concentrations of corticosteroids in the posterior eye, and a reduction in adverse effects compared to systemic administration. Intraocular levels of corticosteroids are identical between subtenon and retrobulbar administration [102]. For oral administration, the initial high dose ($1-1.5\,\mathrm{mg\,kg^{-1}}$) is subsequently decreased according to clinical effect [22, 34, 91]. Recent publications suggest that the intravitreal application of triamcinolone seems to be a promising therapeutic method for macular edema that fails to respond to conventional treatment [53, 73]. Martidis et al. published a prospective, noncomparative, interventional case series to determine if intravitreal injection of triamcinolone acetonide is safe and effective in treating diabetic macular edema unresponsive to prior laser photocoagulation [73]. Sixteen eyes with clinically significant diabetic macular edema (CSME) that failed to respond to at least two previous sessions of laser photocoagulation were included in the study. The response of the laser treatment was measured by clinical examination and optical coherence tomography (OCT) at least six months after initial laser therapy. Eyes with a residual central macular thickness of more than $300\,\mu\mathrm{m}$ (normal: $200\,\mu\mathrm{m}$) and visual loss from baseline were offered an intravitreal injection of 4 mg triamcinolone acetonide. In this study, the mean improvement in visual acuity measured 2.4, 2.4, and 1.3 Snellen lines at the one-, three-, and six-month follow-up intervals, respectively. The central macular thickness as measured by OCT decreased by 55, 57.5, and 38%, respectively, over these same intervals from an initial pretreatment mean of 540.3 µm (±96.3 µm). Intraocular pressure exceeded 21 mmHg in five, three, and one eye(s), respectively, during these intervals. One eye exhibited cataract progression at six months. No other complications were noted over a mean follow-up of 6.2 months. Reinjection was performed in three of eight eyes after six months because of recurrence of macular edema. Similar pilot studies were performed in patients with uveitis, central vein occlusion, and cystoid macular edema after cataract surgery [6, 39, 53, 112]. In most published reports, complications do not appear to be prohibitive; however, all reports demonstrate a limited number of selected cases.

Further randomized studies are therefore warranted to assess long-term efficacy and the need for retreatment. Preliminary data from Jonas et al. suggest that there is no tachyphylaxis in visual acuity or intraocular pressure outcomes after repeated intravitreal injections of triamcinolone acetonide [54].

Upon reviewing the published data on intravitreal injections of triamcinolone acetonide, the therapeutic window seems very wide. The dose range of intravitreally injected triamcinolone acetonide varies from 2 mg [6] to 4 mg [73, 112] and even 25 mg in a single report [51]. Interestingly, reaccumulation of fluid in cystoid spaces occurs between six weeks and three months after injection, and this does not seem to be dose-dependent. Repeated injections at intervals ranging from ten weeks [52] to more than six months [6] show a variable treatment response. There are currently no data on the pharmacokinetic profile of intravitreal triamcinolone, which might be altered after previous vitrectomy. Physiologic intravitreal cortisol levels are reported to be 5.1 ng ml^{-1}, and vitreous levels after peribulbar injections are in the range of 13 mg ml^{-1}. The effective dose of the triamcinolone acetonide is further influenced by the mandatory washes of the widely used stabilizing agent benzylethanol during the preparation of the injection that, even if standardized, alter the remaining amounts of the drug in the solution. Additionally, an inhibitory effect of the stabilizing agent on the drug cannot be excluded. Jaffe and coworkers [49, 50] constructed a fluocinolone acetonide drug delivery device that releases fluocinolone acetonide in a linear manner over an extended period. A clinical phase III study by Bausch & Lomb investigated the efficacy of 0.5 mg (slow-release) fluocinolone acetonide in 80 patients with diffuse diabetic macular edema. Patients receiving the implant showed a statistically significant regression of retinal thickness after six months in comparison to the control group. Furthermore, 80%

of the eyes in the treatment group demonstrated a stable or improved visual acuity compared to only 50% of the eyes of the control group.

Elevation of the intraocular pressure after triamcinolone acetonide of more than 5 mmHg has been reported in up to 30% of eyes [110]. It is therefore prudent to ask patients about any history of steroid response. The incidence of culture-positive endophthalmitis following intravitreal triamcinolone was as rare as 0.87% in a large, multicenter, retrospective case series [80]. Roth and coworkers reported on seven patients who developed a clinical picture simulating endophthalmitis following intravitreal triamcinolone injection [93]. Extensive signs of inflammation developed 1–2 days after injection, at an earlier time point than in bacterial endophthalmitis. Vitreous taps were sterile and inflammation resolved spontaneously, with recovery to preinjection visual acuity or better. This inflammatory response might be a response to the stabilizing additive benzylethanol (see above). In any case, it is recommended that a sterile protocol for intravitreal injections of triamcinolone acetonide should be followed.

Figures 4.1 and 4.2 show the efficacy of intravitreal triamcinolone in a patient with diffuse diabetic macula edema.

4.4.3 Antiangiogenic Treatment

As discussed above, anti-VEGF therapies are closely related to the modification of inflammatory mechanisms in DR.

Currently, there are three VEGF inhibitors that are commonly used in the treatment of proliferative retinopathies and age-related macular degeneration: pegaptanib (Macugen, OSI/Eyetech), bevacizumab (Avastin, Genentech), and ranibizumab (Lucentis, Genentech). While both pegaptanib and ranibizumab are approved for neovascular age-related macular degeneration in the US and many European countries, neither of the agents is yet approved for the treatment of diabetes-related eye disease. Both pegaptanib and ranibizumab are currently under investigation in prospective clinical trials for the treatment of DR.

4.4.3.1 Phase 2 Trial: Intravitreous Pegaptanib as a Treatment for DME

Pegaptanib was evaluated in a randomized, sham-controlled, double-masked, dose-ranging, multicenter phase 2 trial which enrolled 172 patients of 18 years or older with type I or type II diabetes, a visual acuity (VA)

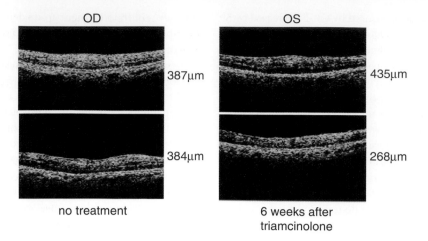

Fig. 4.1 Optical coherence tomography of diabetic macula edema before and after the injection of 4 mg triamcinolone acetonide. There is a significant reduction in retinal thickness

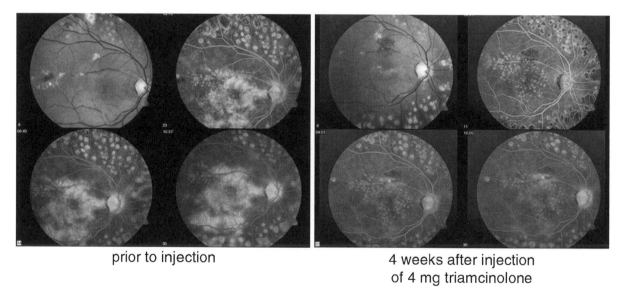

Fig. 4.2 Fluorescein angiography in a patient with diabetic macula edema demonstrating diffuse leakage in the late-phase angiogram. After injection of triamcinolone acetonide, laser scars become visible and there is a large reduction in vascular leakage

of between 20/50 and 20/320, and with DME affecting the center of the macula [23]. Patients were randomized to four treatment arms (0.3 mg, 1 mg, 3 mg pegaptanib or sham injection), with stratification by study site, size of the thickened retina area (≤2.5 disc areas vs. >2.5 disc areas), and baseline VA (ETDRS letter score ≥58 vs. <58). Injections were given at baseline and every six weeks thereafter for a minimum of three from baseline to week 12. Additional injections to a total maximum of six injections were allowed at the investigator's discretion from weeks 18 to 30. Focal/grid laser photocoagulation was also allowed at the investigator's discretion after week 12.

Main efficacy assessments were made at week 36, or six weeks after the last injection.

Pegaptanib treatment was superior to sham injection, according to all prespecified endpoints. Mean change in VA in the 0.3 mg pegaptanib-treated group was +4.7 letters, compared to −0.4 letters for sham ($P = 0.04$). Pegaptanib treatment also resulted in more patients gaining ≥0, ≥5, ≥10, and ≥15 letters of VA. Mean change in center point (foveal) retinal thickness was −68 micrometers in the 0.3 mg pegaptanib arm, compared to +3.7 micrometers in the sham group ($P = 0.02$) and pegaptanib treatment resulted in significantly more patients experiencing decreases in thickness of ≥ 75 and ≥ 100 micrometers). Also, macular volume decreased $0.58\,mm^3$ in the 0.3 mg pegaptanib arm, but increased $0.12\,mm^3$ with sham ($P = 0.009$) (data on file, (OSI) Eyetech, Inc. and Pfizer Inc. 2005). OCT center point thickness at baseline and change in thickness from baseline to week 36 had a modest correlation with VA at baseline or change in VA from baseline to week 36 ($R^2 = 0.18$). Lastly, in the 0.3 mg pegaptanib arm, only 25% of patients required further treatment with photocoagulation, compared to 48% in the sham group ($P = 0.042$) [23].

Fundus photographs were graded in a masked fashion for the presence of neovascularization. A retrospective analysis was done to evaluate the effects of pegaptanib on retinal neovascularization. Nineteen patients in all were found to have retinal revascularization in the study eye, 16 of whom were available for full analysis. Thirteen patients had received pegaptanib while the other three received sham injections. Four of the 13 pegaptanib-treated patients also had neovascularization in the fellow eye. At 36 weeks, eight of the 13 patients in the pegaptanib groups (61%) showed regression of neovascularization, as assessed by fundus photography, while no regression was seen in the three sham-treated patients, or in the four fellow eyes. Three of the eight patients with regressed neovascularization experienced a recurrence between weeks 36 and 52, after pegaptanib therapy was discontinued [2].

4.4.3.2 Clinical Experience with Bevacizumab in Diabetic Retinopathy

Several published studies have demonstrated a biological effect of intravitreal bevacizumab in proliferative diabetic retinopathy and diabetic macular edema. The majority of these studies are limited by their retrospective nature and short follow-up period.

Avery and colleagues retrospectively evaluated the use of intravitreal bevacizumab in patients with retinal neovascularization due to proliferative diabetic retinopathy [10]. In 44 eyes treated with intravitreal bevacizumab ($6.2\,\mu g$ to 1.25 mg), retinal neovascularization demonstrated on fluorescein angiography had complete (or at least partial) reduction in leakage within one week after the injection. Complete resolution of angiographic leakage from neovascularization of the disc was noted in 19 of 26 (73%) eyes, and leakage of iris neovascularization completely resolved in nine of 11 (82%) eyes. The leakage was noted to diminish as early as 24 h after injection. Recurrence of fluorescein leakage varied and was seen as early as two weeks in one case, whereas in other cases, no recurrent leakage was noted at the last available follow-up of 11 weeks. No ocular or systemic adverse events were noted.

Retrospective case series of bevacizumab as an adjunct for intraoperative use in diabetic tractional retinal detachment repair [18] or in eyes with proliferative retinopathy and nonclearing vitreous hemorrhage [100] have been reported. Similarly, intracameral injection of bevacizumab for iris rubeosis [40, 98] has been noted to have a beneficial short-term effect. Although there was a regression of the rubeotic vessels present as early as one week after injection, no persistent effect on intraocular pressure in cases of neovascular glaucoma is yet proven.

In a prospective, consecutive, noncomparative case series, 51 consecutive patients (26 females and 25 males; mean age: 64 years) with diffuse diabetic macular edema were treated with intravitreal bevacizumab [42]. Inclusion criteria were determined independently of the size of edema, retinal thickness, visual acuity, age, metabolic control, type of diabetes, or previous treatments beyond a six-month period. All patients had undergone previous treatments. Sixteen patients (70%) received at least two intravitreal injections of bevacizumab during the study period. Mean central retinal thickness by optical coherence tomography was $501\,\mu m$ (range: $252–1,031\,\mu m$) at baseline and decreased to $425\pm 180\,\mu m$ at two weeks ($P = 0.002$) after bevacizumab, $416\pm 180\,\mu m$ at six weeks ($P = 0.001$), and $377\pm 117\,\mu m$ at 12 weeks ($P = 0.001$). Visual acuity, as measured by ETDRS letters, did not improve significantly through the follow-up period.

A phase II randomized multicenter clinical trial of intravitreal bevacizumab for diabetic macular edema was performed by the Diabetic Retinopathy Clinical Research Network (DRCR.net) [21]. This study involved 121 eyes from 121 individuals with diabetic macular edema involving the center of the macula based on clinical examination, best-corrected Snellen visual acuity equivalent ranging from 20/32 to 20/320, OCT central subfield thickness (CST) greater than or equal to $275\,\mu m$, and no history of treatment for DME in the prior three months. Of the 121 subjects, 109 met criteria for inclusion in the analyses. Subjects were randomized to one of five treatment groups, with 19–24 subjects per group: (a) focal laser photocoagulation at baseline, (b) intravitreal injection of 1.25 mg of bevacizumab at baseline and six weeks, (c) intravitreal injection of 2.5 mg of bevacizumab at baseline and six weeks, (d) intravitreal injection of 1.25 mg of bevacizumab at baseline and sham injection at six weeks, or (e) intravitreal injection of 1.25 mg of bevacizumab at baseline and six weeks with focal photocoagulation at three weeks. Follow-up visits were performed at 3, 6, 9, 12, 18, 24, 41, and 70 weeks. In the 12-week time-frame, there was not a large difference in effect between the two doses of bevacizumab. Interestingly, the reduction in retinal thickness associated with bevacizumab at three weeks appeared to plateau or decrease in most eyes between the three- and six-week visits, suggesting that six weeks might be too long for an optimal initial injection interval. A similar phenomenon was observed after the second injection of bevacizumab. Combining photocoagulation with bevacizumab did not result in any apparent short-term benefit.

This study therefore indicates a short-term response in reduction of retinal thickness from bevacizumab injection. Definitive determinations of a clinically meaningful benefit of intravitreal bevacizumab for DME will require a large phase III randomized clinical trial. This will also be required to provide definitive conclusions regarding safety. No significant safety concerns have arisen to date, but most of the published data on bevacizumab and diabetic eye disease is limited to retrospective case series and anecdotal case reports.

4.4.3.3   Ranibizumab in Diabetic Macula Edema

Nguyen and colleagues conducted an open-label study (Ranibizumab for Edema of the mAcula in Diabetes: A Phase 1 Study—the READ-1 Study) to investigate the effect of intravitreal injections of ranibizumab in patients with DME [83]. Intraocular injections of 0.5 mg of ranibizumab were administered at study entry and at one, two, four, and six months after entry. The injection regimen was selected to assess the effect of three monthly injections and then determine the impact of increasing the time interval between injections to two months for the last two injections. The primary outcome measure was foveal thickness measured by optical coherence tomography (OCT) at seven months compared to baseline.

Among the ten subjects, mean and median visual acuities were better than those at baseline throughout each study time point. At the primary endpoint (seven months after the initial ranibizumab injection), mean and median visual acuity improved by 12.3 and 11 letters in the initial ten subjects, which represents an improvement of a little more than two lines. There was a strong correlation ($R^2 = 0.78$) between visual acuity and foveal thickness as measured by OCT.

The READ-2 Study, a multicenter phase 2 randomized clinical trial investigating the bioactivity and safety of ranibizumab for diabetic macular edema, is underway in the United States. The three treatment arms in the study include: (1) ranibizumab, (2) ranibizumab with focal laser photocoagulation, and (3) focal laser photocoagulation with deferred ranibizumab. Preliminary results are expected in 2008.

Another clinical trial investigating ranibizumab for diabetic retinopathy is also underway, A double-masked, multicenter, phase II study assessing the safety and efficacy of ranibizumab (0.3 and 0.5 mg intravitreal injections) compared with nontreatment control (sham injection) for the treatment of diabetic macular edema is recruiting patients in the United States as well as in Europe, New Zealand and Asia.

Finally, the Diabetic Retinopathy Clinical Research Network (DRCR.net) is conducting a randomized, multi-center clinical trial investigating intravitreal ranibizumab or triamcinolone acetonide in combination with laser photocoagulation for diabetic macular edema. This study will include subjects with diabetic macular edema involving the center of the macula (with an OCT central subfield thickness of greater than 250 microns) responsible for visual acuity of 20/32 or worse. The objective is to determine which is a better treatment approach for DME: laser alone; laser combined with intravitreal triamcinolone; laser combined with intravitreal ranibizumab; or intravitreal ranibizumab alone. Patient recruitment for this study began in March 2007. The primary efficacy outcome will be visual acuity at 12 months adjusted for the baseline acuity, with secondary outcomes being the change in the retinal thickening of the central subfield and retinal volume (measured by OCT) as well as the number of injections in the first year. Safety outcomes will include injection-related events, ocular drug-related events, and systemic drug-related events. A European study is currently ongoing.

Summary for the Clinician

While there are still many questions to be answered regarding the underlying events that ultimately lead to vision loss in diabetes, there is evidence for a major contribution from inflammatory phenomena. This is true for both the vascular damage occurring in the diabetic retina and the neovascularization that is induced in response to the ischemia that attends the loss of capillary blood flow. These findings have already been the basis for the demonstrated clinical benefit of pegaptanib (Macugen™) and ranibizumab (Lucentis™), agents that inactivate VEGF. Results from phase 2 clinical studies should provide further information on the efficacy and safety of VEGF inhibitors in diabetic retinopathy. Inhibitors of VEGF will likely play a therapeutic role for the treatment of both diabetic macular edema and proliferative diabetic retinopathy. There is every reason to expect that further benefits may be seen when other components which regulate these inflammatory events, such as ICAM-1, CD18, TNF- and the Fas/FasL-mediated apoptosis pathway, are similarly targeted.

References

1. Adamis AP, Miller JW, Bernal MT, D'Amico DJ, Folkman J, Yeo TK, Yeo KT (1994) Increased vascular endothelial growth factor levels in the vitreous of eyes with proliferative diabetic retinopathy. Am J Ophthalmol 118:445–450

2. Adamis AP, Altaweel M, Bressler NM, Cunningham ET Jr, Davis MD, Goldbaum M, Gonzales C, Guyer DR, Barrett K, Patel M, Macugen Diabetic Retinopathy Study Group (2006) Changes in retinal neovascularization after pegaptanib (Macugen) therapy in diabetic individuals. Ophthalmology 113:23–28

3. Aiello LP, Avery RL, Arrigg PG, Keyt BA, Jampel HD, Shah ST, Pasquale LR, Thieme H, Iwamoto MA, Park JE, Nguyen HV, Aiello LM, Ferrara N, King GL (1994) Vascular endothelial growth factor in ocular fluid of patients with diabetic retinopathy and other retinal disorders. N Engl J Med 331:1480–1487

4. Aiello LP, Northrup JM, Keyt BA, Takagi H, Iwamoto MA (1995) Hypoxic regulation of vascular endothelial growth factor in retinal cells. Arch Ophthalmol 113:1538–1544

5. Alon T, Hemo I, Itin A, Pe'er J, Stone J, Keshet E (1995) Vascular endothelial growth factor acts as a survival factor for newly formed retinal vessels and has implications for retinopathy of prematurity. Nat Med 1:1024–1028

6. Antcliff RJ, Spalton DJ, Stanford MR, Graham EM, Ffytche TJ, Marshall J (2001) Intravitreal triamcinolone for uveitic cystoid macular edema: an optical coherence tomography study. Ophthalmology 108:765–772

7. Antonetti D, Barber AJ, Hollinger LA, Wolpert EB, Gardner TW (1999) Vascular endothelial growth factor induces rapid phosphorylation of tight junction proteins occludin and zonula occluden 1. J Biol Chem 274:23463–23467

8. Antonetti DA, Wolpert EB, DeMaio L, Harhaj NS, Scaduto RC Jr (2002) Hydrocortisone decreases retinal endothelial cell water and solute flux coincident with increased content and decreased phosphorylation of occludin. J Neurochem 80:667–677

9. Asahara T, Takahashi T, MasudaH, Kalka C, Chen D, Iwaguro H, Inai Y, Silver M, Isner JM (1999) VEGF contributes to postnatal neovascularization by mobilizing bone marrow-derived endothelial progenitor cells. EMBO J 18:3964–3972

10. Avery RL, Pearlman J, Pieramici DJ, Rabena MD, Castellarin AA, Nasir MA, Giust MJ, Wendel R, Patel A (2006) Intravitreal bevacizumab (Avastin) in the treatment of proliferative diabetic retinopathy. Ophthalmology 113(10;1695):E1–E15

11. Barleon B, Sozzani S, Zhou D, Weich HA, Mantovani A, Marme D (1996) Migration of human monocytes in response to vascular endothelial growth factor (VEGF) is mediated via the VEGF receptor flt-1. Blood 87:3336–3343

12. Blaauwgeers HG, Holtkamp GM, Rutten H, Witmer AN, Koolwijk P, Partanen TA, et al. (1999) Polarized vascular endothelial growth factor secretion by human retinal pigment epithelium and localization of vascular endothelial growth factor receptors on the inner choriocapillaris. Evidence for a trophic paracrine relation. Am J Pathol 155:421–428

13. Boeri D, Cagliero E, Podesta F, Lorenzi M (1994) Vascular wall von Willebrand factor in human diabetic retinopathy. Invest Ophthalmol Vis Sci 35:600–607

14. Bresnick GH (1986) Diabetic macular edema. A review. Ophthalmology 93:989–997

15. Brooks HL Jr, Caballero S Jr, Newell CK, Steinmetz RL, Watson D, Segal MS, Harrison JK, Scott EW, Grant MB (2004) Vitreous levels of vascular endothelial growth factor and stromal-derived factor 1 in patients with diabetic retinopathy and cystoid macular edema before and after intraocular injection of triamcinolone. Arch Ophthalmol 122:1801–1807

16. Brown PO, Botstein D (1999) Exploring the new world of the genome with DNA microarrays. Nat Genet 21:S33–S37

17. Caldwell RB, Bartoli M, Behzadian MA, El-Remessy AE, Al-Shabrawey M, Platt DH, Caldwell RW (2003) Vascular endothelial growth factor and diabetic retinopathy: pathophysiological mechanisms and treatment perspectives. Diabetes Metab Res Rev 19:442–455

18. Chen E, Park CH (2006) Use of intravitreal bevacizumab as a preoperative adjunct for tractional retinal detachment repair in severe proliferative diabetic retinopathy. Retina 26:699–700

19. Clauss M, Gerlach M, Gerlach H, Brett J, Wang F, Familletti PC, Pan YC, Olander JV, Connolly DT, Stern D (1990) Vascular permeability factor: a tumor-derived polypeptide that induces endothelial cell and monocyte procoagulant activity, and promotes monocyte migration. J Exp Med 172:1535–1545

20. Comer GM, Ciulla TA (2004) Pharmacotherapy for diabetic retinopathy. Curr Opin Ophthalmol 15:508–518

21. Diabetic Retinopathy Clinical Research Network (2007) A phase 2 randomized clinical trial of intravitreal bevacizumab for diabetic macular edema. Ophthalmology 114:1860–1867

22. Cunningham ET Jr, Adamis AP, Altaweel M, Aiello LP, Bressler NM, D'Amico DJ, Goldbaum M, Guyer DR, Katz B, Patel M, Schwartz SD, Macugen Diabetic Retinopathy Study Group (2005) A phase II randomized double-masked trial of pegaptanib, an anti-vascular endothelial growth factor aptamer, for diabetic macular edema. Ophthalmology 112:1747–1757

23. Dick AD (1994) The treatment of chronic uveitic macular edema. Br J Ophthalmol 78:1–2

24. Duggan DJ, Bittner M, Chen Y, Meltzer P, Trent JM (1999) Expression profiling using cDNA microarrays. Nat Genet 21:S10–S14

4

25. Engerman RL, Kern TS (1995) Retinopathy in galactosemic dogs continues to progress after cessation of galactosemia. Arch Ophthalmol 113:355–358

26. Espinosa-Heidmann DG, Suner IJ, Hernandez EP, Monroy D, Csaky KG, Cousins SW (2003) Macrophage depletion diminishes lesion size and severity in experimental choroidal neovascularization. Invest Ophthalmol Vis Sci 44: 3586–3592

27. Early Treatment Diabetic Retinopathy Study Research Group (1985) Photocoagulation for diabetic macular edema. Early Treatment Diabetic Retinopathy Study Report Number 1. Arch Ophthalmol 103:1796–1806

28. ETDRS Investigators (1992) Aspirin effects on mortality and morbidity in patients with diabetes mellitus. ETDRS Report No. 14. JAMA 268:1292–1300

29. Famiglietti EV, Stopa EG, McGookin ED, Song P, LeBlanc V, Streeten BW (2003) Immunocytochemical localization of vascular endothelial growth factor in neurons and glial cells of human retina. Brain Res 969:195–204

30. Ferrara N (2004) Vascular endothelial growth factor: basic science and clinical progress. Endocr Rev 25:581–611

31. Ferris FL 3rd, Patz A (1984) Macular edema. A complication of diabetic retinopathy. Surv Ophthalmol 28(Suppl):452–461

32. Fong DS, Aiello LP, Ferris FL 3rd, Klein R (2004) Diabetic retinopathy. Diabetes Care 27:2540–2553

33. Franks WA, Limb GA, Stanford MR, Ogilvie J, Wolstencroft RA, Chignell AH, Dumonde DC (1992) Cytokines in human intraocular inflammation. Curr Eye Res 11:187–191

34. Freeman G (2001) Cystoid macular oedema in uveitis: an unsolved problem. Eye 15:12–17

35. Funatsu H, Yamashita H, Shimizu E, Kojima R, Hori S (2001) Relationship between vascular endothelial growth factor and interleukin-6 in diabetic retinopathy. Relationship between vascular endothelial growth factor and interleukin- 6 in diabetic retinopathy. Retina 21:469–477

36. Funatsu H, Yamashita H, Ikeda T, Nakanishi Y, Kitano S, Hori S (2002) Angiotensin II and vascular endothelial growth factor in the vitreous fluid of patients with diabetic macular edema and other retinal disorders. Am J Ophthalmol 133:537–543

37. Funatsu H, Yamashita H, Sakata K, Noma H, Mimura T, Suzuki M, Eguchi S, Hori S (2005) Vitreous levels of vascular endothelial growth factor and intercellular adhesion molecule 1 are related to diabetic macular edema. Ophthalmology 112:806–816

38. Gardiner TA, Gibson DS, de Gooyer TE, de la Cruz VF, McDonald DM, Stitt AW (2005) Inhibition of tumor necrosis factor-alpha improves physiological angiogenesis and reduces pathological neovascularization in ischemic retinopathy. Am J Pathol 166:637–644

39. Greenberg PB, Martidis A, Rogers AH, Duker JS, Reichel E (2002) Intravitreal triamcinolone acetonide for macular oedema due to central retinal vein occlusion. Br J Ophthalmol 86:247–248

40. Grisanti S, Biester S, Peters S, Tatar O, Ziemssen F, Bartz-Schmidt KU, Tuebingen Bevacizumab Study Group (2006) Intracameral bevacizumab for iris rubeosis. Am J Ophthalmol 142:158–160

41. Grossniklaus HE, Ling JX, Wallace TM, Dithmar S, Lawson DH, Cohen C, et al. (2002) Macrophage and retinal pigment epitheliumexpression of angiogenic cytokines in choroidal neovascularization. Mol Vis 8:119–126

42. Haritoglou C, Kook D, Neubauer A, Wolf A, Priglinger S, Strauss R, Gandorfer A, Ulbig M, Kampik A (2006) Intravitreal bevacizumab (Avastin) therapy for persistent diffuse diabetic macular edema. Retina 26:999–1005

43. Hangai M, He S, Hoffmann S, Lim JI, Ryan SJ, Hinton DR (2006) Sequential induction of angiogenic growth factors by TNF-alpha in choroidal endothelial cells. J Neuroimmunol 171:45–56

44. Hawrami K, Hitman GA, Rema M, Snehalatha C, Viswanathan M, Ramachandran A, Mohan V (1996) An association in non-insulin-dependent diabetes mellitus subjects between susceptibility to retinopathy and tumor necrosis factor polymorphism. Hum Immunol 46:49–54

45. Ishida S, YamashiroK, UsuiT, KajiY, Ogura Y, Hida T, Honda Y, Oguchi Y, Adamis AP (2003) Leukocytes mediate retinal vascular remodeling during development and vasoobliteration in disease. Nat Med 9:781–788

46. Ishida S, Usui T, YamashiroK, KajiY, Ahmed E, Carrasquillo KG, et al. (2003) Vegf164 is proinflammatory in the diabetic retina. Invest Ophthalmol Vis Sci 44:2155–2162

47. Ishida S, Usui T, Yamashiro K, Kaji Y, Amano S, Ogura Y, Hida T, Oguchi Y, Ambati J, Miller JW, Gragoudas ES, Ng YS, D'Amore PA, Shima DT, Adamis AP (2003) VEGF164-mediated inflammation is required for pathological, but not physiological, ischemia-induced retinal neovascularization. J Exp Med 198:483–489

48. Iyer VR, Eisen MB, Ross DT, Schuler G, Moore T, Lee JCF, Trent M, Staudt LM, Hudson JJ, Boguski MS, Lashkari DL, Shalon D, Botstein D, Brown PO (1999) The transcriptional program in response of human fibroblasts to serum. Science 293:83–87

49. Jaffe GJ, Ben-Nun J, Guo H, Dunn JP, Ashton P (2000) Fluocinolone acetonide sustained drug delivery device to treat severe uveitis. Ophthalmology 107:2024–2033

50. Jaffe GJ, Yang CH, Guo H, Denny JP, Lima C, Ashton P (2000) Safety and pharmacokinetics of an intraocular fluocinolone acetonide sustained delivery device. Invest Ophthalmol Vis Sci 41:3569–3575

51. Jonas JB, Sofker A (2001) Intraocular injection of crystalline cortisone as adjunctive treatment of diabetic macular edema. Am J Ophthalmol 132:425–427

52. Jonas JB, Kreissig I, Degenring RF (2002) Intravitreal triamcinolone acetonide as treatment of macular edema

in central retinal vein occlusion. Graefes Arch Clin Exp Ophthalmol 240:782–783

53. Jonas JB, Kreissig I, Sofker A, Degenring RF (2003) Intravitreal injection of triamcinolone for diffuse diabetic macular edema. Arch Ophthalmol 121:57–61

54. Jonas JB, Spandau UH, Kamppeter BA, Vossmerbaeumer U, Harder B, Sauder G (2006) Repeated intravitreal high-dosage injections of triamcinolone acetonide for diffuse diabetic macular edema. Ophthalmology 113:800–804

55. Joussen AM, Huang S, Poulaki V, Camphausen K, Beecken WD, Kirchhof B, Adamis AP (2001) In vivo retinal gene expression in early diabetes. Invest Ophthalmol Vis Sci 42:3047–3057

56. Joussen AM, Murata T, Tsujikawa A, Kirchhof B, Bursell SE, Adamis AP (2001) Leukocyte-mediated endothelial cell injury and death in the diabetic retina. Am J Pathol 158:147–152

57. Joussen AM, Poulaki V, Mitsiades N, Kirchhof B, Koizumi K, Dohmen S, Adamis AP (2002) Potential use of non-steroidal anti-inflammatory drugs for prevention of diabetic vascular changes: Aspirin prevents diabetic leakage and leukocyte adhesion through inhibition of TNF-a. FASEB J 16:438–440

58. Joussen AM, Poulaki V, Qin W, Kirchhof B, Mitsiades N, Wiegand SJ, Rudge J, Yancopoulos GD, Adamis AP (2002) Retinal vascular endothelial growth factor induces intercellular adhesionmolecule-1 and endothelial nitric oxide synthase expression and initiates early diabetic retinal leukocyte adhesion in vivo. Am J Pathol 160:501–509

59. Joussen AM, Qin W, Poulaki V, Wiegand S, Yancopoulos GD, Adamis AP (2002) Endogenous VEGF induces retinal ICAM-1 and eNOS expression and initiates early diabetic retinal leukostasis. Am J Pathol 160:501–509

60. Joussen AM, Poulaki V, Mitsiades N, Cai WY, Suzuma I, Pak J, Ju ST, Rook SL, Esser P, Mitsiades CS, Kirchhof B, Adamis AP, Aiello LP (2003) Suppression of Fas-FasL-induced endothelial cell apoptosis prevents diabetic blood-retinal barrier breakdown in a model of streptozotocin-induced diabetes. FASEB J 17:76–78

61. Joussen AM, Poulaki V, Le ML, Koizumi K, Esser C, Janicki H, Schraermeyer U, Kociok N, Fauser S, Kirchhof B, Kern TS, Adamis AP (2004) A central role for inflammation in the pathogenesis of diabetic retinopathy. FASEB J 18:1450–1452

62. Kern TS, Engerman RL (1995) Galactose-induced retinal microangiopathy in rats. Invest Ophthalmol Vis Sci 36:490–496

63. Kern TS, Engerman RL (1996) A mouse model of diabetic retinopathy. Arch Ophthalmol 114:986–990

64. Khosla PK, Seth V, Tiwari HK, Saraya AK (1982) Effect of aspirin on platelet aggregation in diabetes mellitus. Diabetologia 23(2):104–117

65. Klein R, Klein BE, Moss SE, Cruickshanks KJ (1993) Wisconsin epidemiologic study of diabetic retinopathy. XV. The long term incidence of macular edema. Ophthalmology 102:7–16

66. Klein R, Klein BE, Moss SE, Cruickshanks KJ (1998) The Wisconsin Epidemiologic Study of Diabetic Retinopathy: XVII. The 14-year incidence and progression of diabetic retinopathy and associated risk factors in type 1 diabetes. Ophthalmology 105:1801–1815

67. Kucia M, Jankowski K, Reca R, Wysoczynski M, Bandura L, Allendorf DJ, Zhang J, Ratajczak J, Ratajczak MZ (2004) CXCR4-SDF-1 signalling, locomotion, chemotaxis and adhesion. J Mol Histol 35:233–245

68. Leung DW, Cachianes G, Kuang WJ, Goeddel DV, Ferrara N (1989) Vascular endothelial growth factor is a secreted angiogenic mitogen. Science 246:1306–1309

69. Lim JW, Kim H, Kim KH (2001) Nuclear factor-kappaB regulates cyclooxygenase-2 expression and cell proliferation in human gastric cancer cells. Lab Invest 81:349–360

70. Limb GA, Chignell AH, Green W, LeRoy F, Dumonde DC (1996) Distribution of TNF alpha and its reactive vascular adhesion molecules in fibrovascular membranes of proliferative diabetic retinopathy. Br J Ophthalmol 80:168–173

71. Limb GA, Hickman-Casey J, Hollified RD, Chignell AH (1999) Vascular adhesion molecules in vitreous from eyes with proliferative diabetic retinopathy. Invest Ophthalmol Vis Sci 40:2453–2457

72. Limb GA, Webster L, Soomro H, Janikoun S, Shilling J (1999) Platelet expression of tumour necrosis factor-alpha (TNF-alpha), TNF receptors and intercellular adhesion molecule-1 (ICAM-1) in patients with proliferative diabetic retinopathy. Clin Exp Immunol 118:213–218

73. Martidis A, Duker JS, Greenberg PB, Rogers AH, Puliafito CA, Reichel E, Baumal C (2002) Intravitreal triamcinolone for refractory diabetic macular edema. Ophthalmology 109:920–927

74. McCormack K (1998) Roles of COX-1 and COX-2. J Rheumatol 25:2279–2281

75. McLeod DS, Lefer DJ, Merges C, Lutty GA (1995) Enhanced expression of intracellular adhesion molecule-1 and P-selectin in the diabetic human retina and choroid. Am J Pathol 147:642–653

76. Meleth AD, Agron E, Chan CC, Reed GF, Arora K, Byrnes G, Csaky KG, Ferris FL 3rd, Chew EY (2005) Seruminflammatory markers in diabetic retinopathy. Invest Ophthalmol Vis Sci 46:4295–4301

77. Miyamoto K, Hiroshiba N, Tsujikawa A, Ogura Y (1998) In vivo demonstration of increased leukocyte entrapment in retinal microcirculation of diabetic rats. Invest Ophthalmol Vis Sci 39:2190–2194

78. Miyamoto K, Khosrof S, Bursell SE, Moromizato Y, Aiello LP,Ogura Y, Adamis AP (2000) Vascular endothelial growth factor-induced retinal vascular permeability ismediated by intercellular adhesion molecule-1 (ICAM-1). Am J Pathol 156:1733–1739

4

79. Mizutani M, Kern TS, Lorenzi M (1996) Accelerated death of retinal microvascular cells in human and experimental diabetic retinopathy. J Clin Invest 97:2883–2890

80. Moshfeghi DM, Kaiser PK, Scott IU, Sears JE, Benz M, Sinesterra JP, Kaiser RS, Bakri SJ, Maturi RK, Belmont J, Beer PM, Murray TG, Quiroz-Mercado H, Meiler WF (2003) Acute endophthalmitis following intravitreal triamcinolone acetonide injection. Am J Ophthalmol 136:793–796

81. Nagata S, Golstein P (1995) The Fas death factor. Science 267:1449–1456

82. Ng EW, Adamis AP (2005) Targeting angiogenesis, the underlying disorder in neovascular age-related macular degeneration. Can J Ophthalmol 40:352–368

83. Nguyen QD, Tatlipinar S, Shah SM, Haller JA, Quinlan E, Sung J, Zimmer-Galler I, Do DV, Campochiaro PA (2006) Vascular endothelial growth factor is a critical stimulus for diabetic macular edema. Am J Ophthalmol 142(6): 961–969

84. Nishihira J (1998) Novel pathophysiological aspects of macrophage migration inhibitory factor (review). Int J Mol Med 2:17–28

85. Oh H, Takagi H, Takagi C, Suzuma K, Otani A, Ishida K, Matsumura M, Ogura Y, Honda Y (1999) The potential angiogenic role of macrophages in the formation of choroidal neovascular membranes. Invest Ophthalmol Vis Sci 40:1891–1898

86. Pairet M, Engelhardt G (1996) Distinct isoforms (COX-1 and COX-2) of cyclooxygenase: possible physiological and therapeutic implications. Fundam Clin Pharmacol 10:1–17

87. Pillinger MH, Capodici C, Rosenthal P, Kheterpal N, Hanft S, Philips MR, Weissmann G (1998) Modes of action of aspirin-like drugs: salycylates inhibit erk activation and integrin-dependent neutrophil adhesion. Proc Natl Acad Sci USA 95:14540–14545

88. Powell EDU, Field RA (1964) Diabetic retinopathy in rheumatoid arthritis. Lancet 2:17–18

89. Qaum T, Xu Q, Joussen AM, Clemens MW, Qin W, Miyamoto K, Hassessian H, Wiegand SJ, Rudge J, Yancopoulos GD, Adamis AP (2001) VEGF-initiated blood-retinal barrier breakdown in early diabetes. Invest Ophthalmol Vis Sci 42:2408–2413

90. Roberts WG, Palade GE (1995) Increased microvascular permeability and endothelial fenestration induced by vascular endothelial growth factor. J Cell Sci 108:2369–2379

91. Rojas B, Zafirakis P, Christen W, Markomichelakis NN, Foster CS (1999) Medical treatment of macular edema in patients with uveitis. Doc Ophthalmol 97:399–407

92. Romero IA, Radewicz K, Jubin E, Michel CC, Greenwood J, Couraud PO, Adamson P (2003) Changes in cytoskeletal and tight junctional proteins correlate with decreased permeability induced by dexamethasone in cultured rat brain endothelial cells. Neurosci Lett 334:112–116

93. Roth DB, Chieh J, Spirn MJ, Green SN, Yarian DL, Chaudhry NA (2003) Noninfectious endophthalmitis associated with intravitreal triamcinolone injection. Arch Ophthalmol 121:1279–1282

94. Safieh-Garabedian B, Dardenne M, Kanaan SA, Atweh SF, Jabbur SJ, Saade NE (2000) The role of cytokines and prostaglandin-E(2) in thymulin induced hyperalgesia. Neuropharmacology 39:1653–1661

95. Sakane S, Nishihira J, Hirokawa J, Yoshimura H, Honda T, Aoki K, Tagami S, Kawakami Y (1999) Regulation of macrophage migration inhibitory factor (MIF) expression by glucose and insulin in adipocytes in vitro. Mol Med 5:361–371

96. Sakurai E, Anand A, Ambati BK, van Rooijen N, Ambati J (2003) Macrophage depletion inhibits experimental choroidal neovascularization. Invest Ophthalmol Vis Sci 44:3578–3585

97. Sfikakis PP, Markomichelakis N, Theodossiadis GP, Grigoropoulos V, Katsilambros N, Theodossiadis PG (2005) Regression of sight-threatening macular edema in type 2 diabetes following treatment with the anti-tumor necrosis factor monoclonal antibody infliximab. Diabetes Care 28:445–447

98. Silva Paula J, Jorge R, Alves Costa R, Rodrigues Mde L, Scott IU (2006) Short-term results of intravitreal bevacizumab (Avastin) on anterior segment neovascularization in neovascular glaucoma. Acta Ophthalmol Scand 84:556–557

99. Southern E, Mir K, Schepinov M (1999) Molecular interactions on microarrays. Nat Genet 21:S5–S9

100. Spaide RF, Fisher YL (2006) Intravitreal bevacizumab (Avastin) treatment of proliferative diabetic retinopathy complicated by vitreous hemorrhage. Retina 26:275–278

101. Spranger J, Meyer-Schwickerath R, Klein M, Schatz H, Pfeiffer A (1995) TNF-alpha Konzentration in Glaskörper. Anstieg bei neovaskulären Erkrankungen und proliferativer diabetischer Retinopathie. Med Klin 90:134–137

102. Thach AB, Dugel PU, Flindall RJ, Sipperley JO, Sneed SR (1997) A comparison of retrobulbar versus subtenon's corticosteroid therapy for cystoid macular edema refractory to topical medications. Ophthalmology 104:2003–2008

103. Tolentino MJ, Miller JW, Gragoudas ES, Jakobiec FA, Flynn E, Chatzistefanou K, Ferrara N, Adamis AP (1996) Intravitreous injections of vascular endothelial growth factor produce retinal ischemia and microangiopathy in an adult primate. Ophthalmology 103:1820–1828

104. Tsutsumi C, Sonoda KH, Egashira K, Qiao H, Hisatomi T, Nakao S, Ishibashi M, Charo IF, Sakamoto T, Murata T, Ishibashi T (2003) The critical role of ocular-infiltrating macrophages in the development of choroidal neovascularization. J Leukoc Biol 74:25–32

105. Usui T, Ishida S, YamashiroK, Kaji Y, Poulaki V, Moore J, et al. (2004) Vegf 164(165) as the pathological isoform: Differential leukocyte and endothelial responses through vegfr1 and vegfr2. Invest Ophthalmol Vis Sci 45: 368–374

106. Wallach D (1997) Cell death induction by TNF: a matter of self control. Trends Biochem Sci 22:107–109

107. Watanabe D, Suzuma K, Suzuma I, Ohashi H, Ojima T, Kurimoto M, Murakami T, Kimura T, Takagi H (2005) Vitreous levels of angiopoietin 2 and vascular endothelial growth factor in patients with proliferative diabetic retinopathy. Am J Ophthalmol 139:476–481

108. Watanabe D, Suzuma K, Matsui S, Kurimoto M, Kiryu J, Kita M, Suzuma I, Ohashi H, Ojima T, Murakami T, Kobayashi T, Masuda S, Nagao M, Yoshimura N, Takagi H (2005) Erythropoietin as a retinal angiogenic factor in proliferative diabetic retinopathy. N Engl J Med 353: 782–792

109. Weissmann G (1991) Aspirin. Sci Am 264:84–96

110. Wingate RJ, Beaumont PE (1999) Intravitreal triamcinolone and elevated intraocular pressure. Aust NZ J Ophthalmol 27:431–432

111. Yoshikawa K, Kotake S, Ichiishi A, Sasamoto Y, Kosaka S, Matsuda J (1995) Posterior sub-tenon injections of repository corticosteroids in uveitis patients with cystoidmacular edema. Jpn J Ophthalmol 39:71–76

112. Young S, Larkin G, Branley M, Lightman S (2001) Safety and efficacy of intravitreal triamcinolone for cystoid macular oedema in uveitis. Clin Exp Ophthalmol 29:2–6

Chapter 5

Steroid Sensitivity in Uveitis

5

Richard W.J. Lee, Lauren P. Schewitz, Ben J.E. Raveney, Andrew D. Dick

Core Messages

- Endogenous glucocorticoids, under the regulation of the hypothalamic–pituitary–adrenal axis, play a fundamental role in control of the normal immune response
- Glucocorticoids induce both gene upregulation (transactivation) and gene suppression (transrepression)
- Exogenous glucocorticoids remain the first-line treatment for noninfectious uveitis
- Up to a quarter of uveitis patients are refractory to treatment with tolerable glucocorticoid doses

- The problem of suboptimal therapeutic responses to glucocorticoids is generic to a range of inflammatory and lymphoproliferative diseases
- Potentiation of IL-2-mediated effects is a strong candidate mechanism for generating steroid refractory disease
- Future strategies to optimise glucocorticoid efficacy include concomitant use of anti-CD25 monoclonal antibodies target steroid refractory T cells, and the development of novel glucocorticoid receptor ligands

5.1 Introduction

Corticosteroids are the old talisman of immunotherapies. They have revolutionised the treatment of inflammatory, autoimmune, and lymphoproliferative diseases, bringing benefit to many millions of patients. Their continued pre-eminence almost 60 years after the Nobel Prize was awarded for their discovery and use in rheumatoid arthritis [18] is testament to their status as one of the most important drugs in medicine. However, up to a quarter of patients are refractory to treatment and their wide-ranging side-effects have rightly motivated the search for alternative immunosuppressive drugs.

Ophthalmologists have adopted a number of strategies to optimise corticosteroid therapy for ocular inflammatory diseases, principally by utilising local routes of administration to minimise systemic side-effects. Topical, subconjunctival, orbital floor, subtenon and intravitreal delivery are all commonplace, but not without significant cost, as they induce both cataract and glaucoma [6]. Their efficacy is also insufficient to suppress the inflammatory response in idiopathic sight-threatening noninfectious posterior segment intraocular inflammation, or when associated with multisystem inflammatory conditions (e.g. sarcoidosis and Behçets disease). We therefore rely on systemic corticosteroid treatment, often in combination with alternative immunosuppressive agents, such as T cell inhibitors (e.g. cyclosporine and tacrolimus), antimetabolites (e.g. methotrexate and mycophenolate mofetil) and biologics (e.g. anti-TNF-α and interferon-α), to induce and maintain disease remission in the majority of patients with noninfectious ocular inflammatory disease—with varying degrees of success[20].

In this chapter, we review the role of corticosteroids in health and disease, and examine the mechanisms that modulate patient responses to treatment. This is described in the context of emerging therapeutic approaches to combat steroid refractory inflammation and the ongoing search for the panacea of side-effect-free glucocorticoid (GC) immunosuppression.

5.2 Glucocorticoids as Regulators of the Immune Response

5.2.1 Endogenous Glucocorticoids and the Hypothalamic–Pituitary–Adrenal Axis

Cortisol is the principal endogenous corticosteroid. It is released by the adrenal cortex and regulates the immune response through its GC effects. Adrenal cortisol secretion is controlled by adrenocorticotropic hormone (ACTH), which, in turn, is secreted into the general circulation by the anterior pituitary gland under the influence of corticotropin-releasing hormone (CRH) from the hypothalamus. A range of circadian, emotional, neurological, and immune stimuli sit at the top of this physiological hierarchy, reflecting the range of metabolic and immune functions mediated by GCs. Together they comprise the hypothalamic–pituitary–adrenal (HPA) axis, which plays a central role in the normal stress response under the intimate control of a series of negative feedback loops (Fig. 5.1) [39].

GCs have a great diversity of actions in addition to their immune function. Enhanced cardiovascular tone results from potentiation of vasopressor responses, and this combines with an increased circulating volume caused by renal sodium retention to increase blood pressure [45]. Serum concentrations of glucose and cholesterol are elevated by lipolysis of adipose tissue and hepatic gluconeogenesis, for which muscle is also broken down to provide amino acid substrates [10, 30]. Such prioritisation of short-term energy supply is at the expense of nonessential metabolic processes, such as bone mineralization and chondrocyte proliferation in the growth plates of children [39].

Of all the roles GCs play, maintaining immune homeostasis is the most important. They influence the behaviour of all types of immune cells and coordinate a downregulation and cessation of the immune response. This is orchestrated by the HPA axis with such refinement that fluctuations in the levels of circulating GCs, as observed during exercise and circadian rhythms, are associated with changes in lymphocyte cytokine production [47]. Alterations in HPA axis tone have, therefore, unsurprisingly been implicated in autoimmunity. Rodents with blunted HPA axis responses are highly susceptible to the induction of autoimmune disease in comparison to strains with normal HPA axis function, and are used as the basis for laboratory disease models [46]. For example, Lewis rats immunised with myelin basic protein

develop experimental autoimmune encephalomyelitis (EAE), which mimics multiple sclerosis, resulting in transient paralysis. However, if endogenous GC production is interrupted by adrenolectomy, this disease is fatal. In contrast, administration of exogenous GCs through a subcutaneous implant results in complete EAE remission [29]. The relevance of this to immunity is supported first by observations of impaired HPA axis function in rheumatoid arthritis, systemic lupus erythematosis and Sjogren's syndrome, and second by observations that elevated circulating GC concentrations occur during chronic stress responses, and are associated with an enhanced susceptibility to viral infection and decreased antibody production after vaccination [46].

This fundamental role of the HPA axis and GCs in immunoregulation is well recognised, but it is easily overlooked amid the hype of new discoveries which promise to revolutionise therapies for allergy, autoimmunity and sepsis [4]. However, there remains the potential to optimise our use of exogenous GC therapies to restore immune balance in inflammatory pathology. This requires an understanding of the reasons for varying GC responses between individuals and also an elucidation of the molecular mechanisms that underlie GC function.

Summary for the Clinician

- Endogenous glucocorticoids, under the regulation of the HPA axis, play a fundamental role in control of the normal immune response
- Glucocorticoids also have a great diversity of metabolic actions, including the release of glucose and lipids, the increase of peripheral vascular resistance and demineralisation of bone
- Blunted HPA axis responses predispose to autoimmunity, while chronic HPA overstimulation predisposes to infection
- There is still much potential to optimise glucocorticoid therapy for inflammatory diseases

Fig. 5.1 The control and action of glucocorticoids. Glucocorticoid (GC) secretion is regulated by the HPA axis, although the illustrated mechanisms of action apply whether GC origin is exogenous or endogenous. *Solid lines* represent pathways of action and broken lines represent pathways of inhibition. On entry to the cell, GCs bind to the cytoplasmic GC receptor (GR), which then translocates to the nucleus to either (**A**) inhibit nuclear factor-κB (NFκB) or (**B**) inhibit activator protein 1 (AP-1); both resulting in transcriptional suppression of interleukin-2 (IL-2) as well as other proinflammatory mediators by direct protein–protein interactions (IL-1, TNFα, INFγ). The activated GR also binds to GC response elements in DNA (**C**) and induces the transcription of anti-inflammatory proteins and the inhibitor of κB (IκB) (**D**), resulting in cytosolic retention of NFκB and suppression of its action. In the presence of a T cell response, increased levels of IL-2 engage the IL-2 receptor (IL-2R) (**E**). Signals downstream of the IL-2R then inhibit GR translocation into the nucleus (principally mediated by signal transducer and activator of transcription 5, STAT-5) (**F**) and activate NFκB (**G**), suppressing GC actions. Other abbreviations: *ACTH*, adrenocorticotropic hormone; *CAMs*, cell adhesion molecules; *COX-2*, cyclooxygenase 2; *CRH*, corticotropin-releasing hormone; *GRE*, GC response element; *IFN-γ*, interferon-γ; *IL-1*, interleukin-1; *IL-10*, interleukin-10; *JAK*, Janus kinase; *MAPK*, mitogen-activated protein kinase; *mRNA*, messenger RNA; *p50*, p50 subunit of NFκB; *p65*, p65 subunit of NFκB; *TNF-α*, tumour necrosis factor-α

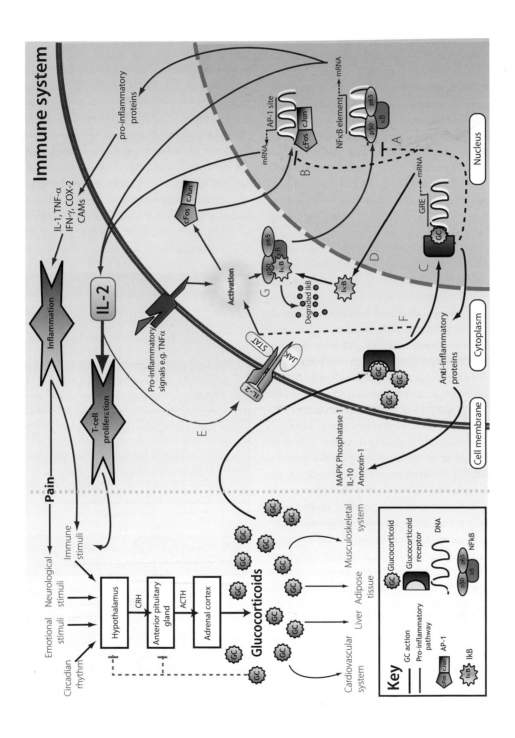

5

5.2.2   Glucocorticoid Control of Cell Function

The immunosuppressive actions of GCs can occur through either genomic or nongenomic mechanisms. GCs enter cells by passive diffusion and bind to their cytosolic glucocorticoid receptor (GR, Fig. 5.1), following which the GC–GR complex translocates into the cell nucleus and associates with specific DNA sequences in the regulatory regions of target genes, resulting in either enhancement or suppression of transcription (either by direct DNA interactions or by indirect interference with other transcription factors, such as nuclear factor-κB (NFκB) and activator protein 1 (AP-1) [40]). Classically, the physiological consequences of GCs were thought to be predominantly due to suppression of gene expression (transrepression), although emerging evidence suggests that gene upregulation (transactivation) plays a greater role [37]. Nongenomic GC mechanisms include the activation of endothelial nitric oxide synthetase (eNOS), resulting in nitric oxide release, which, in combination with GCs, has anti-inflammatory effects [15].

Examples of genomic-mediated immunosuppression via gene transactivation include the induction of annexin 1 (also called lipocortin-1) and mitogen-activated protein kinase (MAPK) phosphatase 1; both of which inhibit the release of arachidonic acid and its subsequent conversion to eicosanoids (e.g. prostaglandins, thromboxanes, prostacyclines and leucotrienes) [39]. As a result of GC-mediated activation of MAPK phosphatase 1, MAPK is deactivated, which further regulates dendritic cell, macrophage and T cell activation, resulting in the suppression and control of immune responses. In addition, the induction of interleukin-10 results in a shift from proinflammatory Th1 T cell-mediated immune responses to anti-inflammatory Th2 T cell-mediated responses [46].

Although transrepression can occur directly via negative GC response elements in DNA, it is mostly mediated through protein–protein interactions between the GR and other transcription factors, particularly AP-1 and NFκB, because of their mutual role in the expression of the T cell growth factor interleukin-2 (IL-2). NFκB also directs the expression of multiple proinflammatory cytokines, such as interleukin-1 (IL-1), TNF-α and interferon-γ (IFN-γ), and contributes to prostaglandin production through induction of cyclooxygenase 2 (COX-2). GCs further antagonize the action of this pivotal proinflammatory transcription factor via the induction of the inhibitor of κB (IκB), and this mechanism is central to the GC suppression of IL-2 production and T cell proliferation [38]. GC-mediated NFκB inhibition also curtails immune cell trafficking via downregulation of cell adhesion molecules, and is key to driving GC-induced apoptosis [46].

5.2.3   The Interleukin-2/Glucocorticoid Balance

The IL-2/GC dynamic is reciprocally regulated. For example, IL-2 in combination with IL-4 has been shown to reduce GR binding affinity and attenuate GC inhibition of T cell proliferation [23]. In addition, IL-2 inhibits GR translocation via signal transducer and activator of transcription 5 (STAT-5) [12]. IL-2 also potentiates the nuclear translocation of Fox03, a forkhead transcription factor responsible for inhibition of the GC-inducible gene glucocorticoid-induced leucine zipper (*gilz*), which mediates GC effects, particularly apoptosis [1]. Hence, the play-off of the cellular effects of competing GC and IL-2 influences is central in determining the balance of the immune response. Concordant with this, there is increasing evidence that IL-2 inhibition of GC action is of key relevance in determining clinical responses to GC therapy [26].

Summary for the Clinician

- Glucocorticoids exert their effects through a combination of gene upregulation (transactivation) and gene suppression (transrepression)
- Transactivation inhibits the release of proinflammatory prostaglandins and induces expression of anti-inflammatory cytokines
- The most important transrepression effect of glucocorticoids is inhibition of NFκB, which results in reduced expression of proinflammatory cytokines, downregulation of immune cell trafficking and increased T cell apoptosis
- These mechanisms are counter-regulated by IL-2, thereby inhibiting glucocorticoid function.

5.3   Glucocorticoids in the Treatment of Noninfectious Uveitis

Exogenous GCs are commonly used for the treatment of noninfectious uveitis. Examples include prednisone and methylprednisolone, both of which have been available since the 1950s. They remain the first-line treatment for ocular inflammation and are the gold standard against which other immunotherapies are judged.

Despite this, there is surprisingly scant evidence supporting the use of systemic GCs in uveitis, with only two prospective, randomised, double-masked trials in cohorts with heterogeneous disease [11, 34]. Both studies were small, with less than 30 patients in each prednisone monotherapy group, and they did not utilise the same GCs regimen (one study used *high-dose* treatment: maximum 80 mg prednisone daily, tapering to 20 mg daily over three months [34]; the other study used *low-dose* treatment: maximum 20 mg prednisone daily, tapering over four months to stop) [11]. Entry criteria were, however, the same and selected for severe disease, with better eye visual acuities (VAs) of 20/40 or worse in association with active inflammation. In the *high-dose* trial, 46% of patients were considered therapeutic successes at three months, defined as a 15-letter improvement in logMAR (logarithm of the minimum angle of resolution) VA or a two-point reduction in vitreous haze. Ten percent of patients were considered therapeutic failures because their logMAR VA reduced by ten letters in the first three months, although the proportion of these in the prednisone group was not reported. In the *low-dose* study, 75% of patients receiving prednisone monotherapy were considered treatment successes when taking 10 mg of prednisone daily, but this dramatically plummeted to a 20% success after prednisone was discontinued. This data is in keeping with clinical experience, i.e. GCs induce disease remission in all but a small minority of refractory patients (who do not respond even to high-dose treatment). However, this benefit is lost on steroid taper, with up to a quarter of patients failing to achieve 10 mg of prednisone daily—and this proportion is even greater in certain uveitic subtypes such as Behçet's [2] and Vogt–Koyanagi–Harada disease [36].

The main limitation of systemic GC therapies is their side effects, which can be directly attributed to their diverse metabolic actions. Water retention and increased peripheral vascular resistance cause hypertension; gluconeogenesis and lipolysis result in secondary diabetes mellitus and hypercholesterolemia; redistribution of adipose tissue and wasting of proximal limb muscles are manifest as a "cushingoid" appearance; bone demineralization causes osteoporosis with an ensuing risk of long bone fracture and vertebral collapse; and inhibition of epiphyseal chondrocytes in children results in growth retardation, which does not fully recover after long-term treatment [39]. The probability of inducing such comorbidity is generally considered to be much reduced in adults at daily prednisone doses of ≤10 mg, and the Standardization of Uveitis Nomenclature Working Group has adopted this threshold as a key measure of treatment efficacy [21]. Hence, additional immunomodulating therapies are frequently used in patients unable to achieve 10 mg prednisone daily, or who follow a relapsing–remitting disease course, to facilitate steroid taper and reduce the frequency of inflammatory reactivations [22].

It is therefore clear that although GCs are the most commonly used immunosuppressive therapy for intraocular inflammation, achieving disease control at tolerable doses remains one of the main challenges for uveitis specialists and their patients. Any new insights into the molecular mechanisms that underlie steroid refractory disease, or the development of new interventions which optimise the immunosuppressive effects of GCs while minimising their side effects, would herald a significant advance.

> ## Summary for the Clinician
>
> - Exogenous glucocorticoids remain the first-line treatment for noninfectious uveitis
> - High-quality clinical evidence supporting their use is limited, but suggests that up to 25% of patients are refractory to tolerable systemic doses (≤10 mg prednisone daily), with a small minority of patients deteriorating despite high-dose treatment
> - The main limitation of current systemic GC therapies is the high incidence of pronounced side effects

5.4 Steroid Sensitivity in Other Inflammatory Diseases

The problem of suboptimal therapeutic responses to GCs and their associated side effects is not isolated to uveitis. In ulcerative colitis (UC), failure to respond to high-dose systemic GCs is an indication for colectomy, and there are validated clinical definitions of steroid resistance [9]. This is estimated to affect up to 30% of patients and represents a considerable burden of disease [44]. Similarly, an important subgroup of asthmatics are refractory to GC treatment with a consequent increased risk of mortality, and considerable effort is currently being directed into improving treatment outcomes for these individuals [3]. In fact, the most difficult patient groups in all GC-treated conditions, in terms of both drug-induced morbidity and poor clinical outcome, are steroid refractory (SR). Notable examples include: SR rheumatoid arthritis [7], SR solid organ allograft rejection [25], SR acute lymphoblastic leukaemia [13], and SR childhood nephrotic syndrome [14]. Hence, although we are currently presenting this issue in the context of uveitis, SR disease represents a major cross-speciality challenge.

5.4.1 The Concept of a Common Steroid Refractory Phenotype

As there is surprisingly little difference in measures of disease severity between steroid responders and nonresponders, and given that up to a third of healthy volunteers have steroid refractory immune responses in vitro, it has been suggested that the SR responses observed clinically across disease groups may have a common underlying phenotype [32]. That is, failure to respond to treatment may be a function of an individual's immune system rather than their disease. SR patients nonetheless suffer GC side effects, so if this concept has credence, the mechanism responsible would have to be immune-specific.

Summary for the Clinician

■ The problem of suboptimal therapeutic responses to glucocorticoids is generic to a range of inflammatory and lymphoproliferative diseases

■ Suboptimal responses are independent of disease severity, and as up to a third of normal volunteers also exhibit steroid refractory (SR) immune responses in vitro, SR disease may simply reflect a common SR phenotype

5.5 Immune Mechanisms of Steroid Resistance

Impaired in vitro responses to the synthetic GC dexamethasone have been observed in peripheral blood mononuclear cells (PBMCs) from patients with SR asthma [8], SR UC [16], SR rheumatoid arthritis [42], SR acute lymphoblastic leukaemia [24], and SR renal transplant recipients [25]. Efforts to identify the cause of this disparity have identified three principal candidate mechanisms: first, enhanced NFκB (and AP-1)-dependent gene expression; second, inhibition of STAT-5-dependent GR translocation into the nucleus; and third, changes in the availability and binding of the GR (particularly a reduced GRα:GRβ ratio; see below). Only the latter is independent of IL-2 upregulation.

The human GR gene is on one locus on chromosome 5q31–32 (Fig. 5.2). There are two exon 9 isoforms that can be spliced to produce mature messenger RNA (mRNA). Splicing of exon 9α produces GRα mRNA, which is translated into a protein with a unique sequence of 50 amino acids at its carboxyl end. This isoform binds GCs, DNA, and other transcription factors, thereby modifying transcriptional activity in target genes. The alternative GRβ mRNA splice variant is translated into a protein with a truncated carboxyl end. Although this is able to bind DNA, it does not bind any ligands and thus fails to activate or suppress transcription. It nonetheless has been shown to form inactive heterodimers with GRα in vitro [39]. Consequently, elevated GRβ levels, as have been observed in SR asthma patients, have a putative role in SR disease [28]. However, this mechanism remains under dispute, as other studies have shown no influence of GRβ on GRα-mediated transactivation and transrepression [17].

Potentiation of IL-2-mediated effects is therefore arguably the prime candidate mechanism for generating

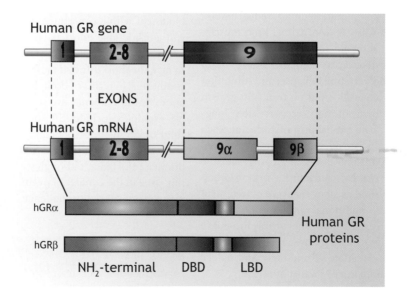

Fig. 5.2 The human glucocorticoid receptor. Exon 9 of the human glucocorticoid receptor (hGR) has two isoforms which can be spliced to produce mature messenger RNA (mRNA). When translated, hGRα has a unique sequence of 50 amino acids at its carboxyl end. *DBD*, DNA-binding domain; *LBD*, ligand-binding domain; *NH₂*, amine

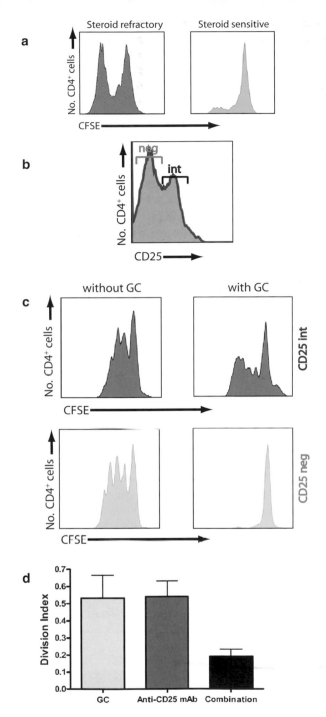

Fig. 5.3 T cell proliferation and cell surface protein expression in response to glucocorticoids and anti-CD25 monoclonal antibodies [26]. **a** CFSE (carboxyfluorescein succinimidyl ester) dilution in CD4$^+$ T cells from a patient with steroid-refractory (SR) ulcerative colitis (*left graph*) and a steroid-sensitive (SS) normal volunteer (*right graph*) after in vitro culture in the presence of high-dose glucocorticoids (GCs). CFSE is a cytoplasmic dye that is equally divided between daughter cells on cell division. Proliferating T cells therefore migrate to the left of the x-axis. The SR patient has a distinct subpopulation of T cells that continue to divide despite the presence of GCs (*left peak*). **b** Expression of CD25 (the α-subunit of the interleukin-2 receptor) in peripheral blood CD4$^+$ T cells. *Neg*, no expression (approx 50% of cells); *Int*, intermediate expression (approx 45% of cells). **c** CFSE dilution in CD4$^+$ CD25^{neg} and CD4$^+$ CD25^{int} cells after in vitro culture in the presence of GCs. CD25^{neg} cells are exquisitely SS, whereas a proportion of CD25^{int} cells are SR. **d** Anti-CD25 monoclonal antibodies (mAb) abrogate proliferation in CD4$^+$ cells escaping GC inhibition in vitro. The "division index" is the average number of divisions each cell has undergone

asthma as compared with those from steroid-sensitive controls [27].

This led to the hypothesis that the SR phenotype is not a feature of all immune cells, but is limited to lymphocytes which express the IL-2 receptor (CD25), and a recent pilot study has identified a subpopulation of SR CD4$^+$ T cells in patients with SR UC (Fig. 5.3a) [26]. This implies a new paradigm for SR disease in which GCs positively select SR cells, generating a subpopulation of lymphocytes which perpetuate ongoing inflammation. SR CD4$^+$ T cells were also shown to express intermediate levels of CD25 (CD25^{int}, Figs. 5.3b, 5.3c), and their continued proliferation in the presence of GCs was abrogated by an anti-CD25 monoclonal antibody (mAb) (Fig. 5.3d) [26], providing corroborative evidence for the importance of IL-2 in modulating GC responses at a cellular level. Analogous investigations to identify a SR subgroup of CD4$^+$ cells in SR uveitis patients are currently underway.

the SR phenotype, and there is accumulating evidence in support of this: IL-2 (with IL-4) reduces both GR binding affinity and GC inhibition of proliferation in PBMCs from normal volunteers to levels seen in PBMCs from SR patients, and it also sustains reduced (albeit reversible) GR affinity in PBMCs from SR patients [23]. Furthermore, IL-2 mRNA expression is significantly greater in bronchoalveolar lavage samples from patients with SR

Summary for the Clinician

- Impaired in vitro immune responses to steroids are consistently observed in patients with steroid refractory (ST) disease
- The main candidate mechanism for this steroid refractory phenotype is an upregulation of IL-2, although an inactive isoform of the glucocorticoid receptor (GRβ) has also been implicated
- Pilot data suggest that SR phenotype is restricted to CD4$^+$ T cells expressing the IL-2 receptor (CD25)

5

5.6 Future Directions: Novel Strategies to Optimise Glucocorticoid Treatment

5.6.1 Targeting Steroid Refractory CD4+ Cd25int Cells

The SR phenotype of CD4+ CD25int T cells makes them a putative target for intervention in the treatment of SR disease. In support of this, a recent Phase II clinical trial of an anti-CD25 mAb has demonstrated clinical rescue in SR ulcerative colitis [9]. The success of calcineurin inhibition with cyclosporine and tacrolimus in the treatment of uveitis also provides indirect evidence that attenuating IL-2 responses translates into improved outcomes for patients with SR ocular inflammation [19, 43]. Of even greater pertinence, however, is the existing Phase I/II trial data evaluating the efficacy of the anti-CD25mAb daclizumab in the treatment of refractory uveitis [33, 35]. In these studies, two small prospective patient cohorts were treated with either 4–6 weekly intravenous (IV) daclizumab infusions ($n = 10$) or two weekly subcutaneous injections ($n = 5$) [33]. All patients were subject to rapid subsequent steroid taper and seven out of the ten patients in the IV study achieved long-term (four-year) treatment success, as did 100% of the subcutaneously treated group (at 26 months). All patients, bar one, were taking systemic steroids when daclizumab was started, the majority at high dose, with only two patients taking less than 10 mg prednisone daily. Of the three patients in the IV study who failed treatment, two maintained disease control for 12 months after starting daclizumab, and one exited after just three months of treatment. As concomitant treatments were discontinued after eight weeks, this implies that all patients in both studies were able to achieve disease remission on a combination of anti-CD25 mAb and prednisone despite being previously treatment-refractory; adding weight to the theory that anti-CD25 therapies potentiate GC effects and abrogate SR disease.

5.6.2 Other Approaches

An alternative approach to augmenting GC action involves the use of selective GR agonists (SEGRAs), which aim to dissociate GC-mediated transrepression (credited with the immunosuppressive effects of GCs) from transactivation (to which the majority of GC side effects are attributed). This is a laudable goal which has attracted considerable pharmaceutical industry interest, with one compound in particular (ZK216348) showing promise in preclinical studies [41]. However, it is probably naïve to expect that the wanted and unwanted effects of GCs are cleanly delineated, as transactivation

also plays an important anti-inflammatory role, and the nongenomic effects of GCs have so far been ignored in drug development [31].

Other attempts to optimise GC efficacy and tolerance have mainly utilised novel means of drug delivery. For example, encapsulating conventional GCs in liposomes, which accumulate selectively at sites of inflammation, and incorporating GCs in timed release tablets [5]. Efforts have also been made to potentiate the action of endogenous GCs by inhibiting their deactivation using 11β-hydroxysteroid dehydrogenase, and to link conventional GCs with nitric oxide to synergise the anti-inflammatory effects of both compounds [5]. Although each has potential, none of these strategies are currently applied in routine clinical practice.

We hope that continued development of novel GC ligands and improved approaches to drug delivery will in the future combine with advances in basic scientific understanding of the molecular mechanisms underlying the SR phenotype to generate therapeutic strategies with sufficient specificity to target SR immune cells, while avoiding unwanted upregulation of GC effects in bystander tissues; thereby overcoming the substantial cross-speciality clinical burden of SR disease and, at last, ensuring that all uveitis patients are steroid-sensitive.

Summary for the Clinician

- CD4+ CD25int T cells are a putative target for therapeutic intervention in steroid refractory disease
- This is supported by successful existing Phase I/II randomised controlled trial data for anti-CD25 monoclonal antibody therapy in refractory uveitis
- Other strategies for optimising steroid sensitivity include improved approaches to drug delivery and the development of novel GR ligands with greater immunosuppressive specificity

---

References

1. Asselin-Labat M-L, Biola-Vidamment A, Kerbrat S, et al. (2005) Fox03 mediates antagonistic effects of glucocorticoids and interleukin-2 on glucocorticoid-induced leucine zipper expression. Mol Endocrinol 19:1752–1764

2. Benezra D, Cohen E, Chajek T, et al. (1988) Evaluation of conventional therapy versus cyclosporine A in Behcet's syndrome. Transplant Proc 20:136–143

3. Berry MA, Hargadon B, Shelley M, et al. (2006) Evidence of a role of tumor necrosis factor {alpha} in refractory asthma. N Engl J Med 354:697–708

4. Besedovsky HO, Del Rey A (2006) Regulating inflammation by glucocorticoids. Nat Immunol 7:537

5. Buttgereit F, Burmester GR, Lipworth BJ (2005) Optimised glucocorticoid therapy: the sharpening of an old spear. Lancet 365:801–803

6. Carnahan MC, Goldstein DA (2000) Ocular complications of topical, peri-ocular, and systemic corticosteroids. Curr Opin Ophthalmol 11:478–483

7. Chikanza IC, Kozaci DL (2004) Corticosteroid resistance in rheumatoid arthritis: molecular and cellular perspectives. Rheumatology 43:1337–1345

8. Corrigan CJ, Brown PH, Barnes NC, et al. (1991) Glucocorticoid resistance in chronic asthma. Glucocorticoid pharmacokinetics, glucocorticoid receptor characteristics, and inhibition of peripheral blood T cell proliferation by glucocorticoids in vitro. Am Rev Respir Dis 144:1016–1025

9. Creed TJ, Norman MR, Probert CS, et al. (2003) Basiliximab (anti-CD25) in combination with steroids may be an effective new treatment for steroid-resistant ulcerative colitis. Aliment Pharmacol Ther 18:65–75

10. Dallman MF, Strack AM, Akana SF, et al. (1993) Feast and famine: critical role of glucocorticoids with insulin in daily energy flow. Front Neuroendocrinol 14:303–347

11. De Vries J, Baarsma GS, Zaal MJ, et al. (1990) Cyclosporin in the treatment of severe chronic idiopathic uveitis. Br J Ophthalmol 74:344–349

12. Goleva E, Kisich KO, Leung DYM (2002) A role for STAT5 in the pathogenesis of IL-2-induced glucocorticoid resistance. J Immunol 169:5934–5940

13. Haarman EG, Kaspers GJ, Veerman AJ (2003) Glucocorticoid resistance in childhood leukaemia: mechanisms and modulation. Br J Haematol 120:919–929

14. Habashy D, Hodson EM, Craig JC (2003) Interventions for steroid-resistant nephrotic syndrome: a systematic review. Pediatr Nephrol 18:906–912

15. Hafezi-Moghadam A, Simoncini T, Yang Z, et al. (2002) Acute cardiovascular protective effects of corticosteroids are mediated by non-transcriptional activation of endothelial nitric oxide synthase. Nat Med 8:473–479

16. Hearing SD, Norman M, Probert CS, et al. (1999) Predicting therapeutic outcome in severe ulcerative colitis by measuring in vitro steroid sensitivity of proliferating peripheral blood lymphocytes. Gut 45:382–388

17. Hecht K, Carlstedt-Duke J, Stierna P, et al. (1997) Evidence that the beta-isoform of the human glucocorticoid receptor does not act as a physiologically significant repressor. J Biol Chem 272:26659–26664

18. Hench PS, Kendall EC, et al. (1949) The effect of a hormone of the adrenal cortex (17-hydroxy-11-dehydrocorticosterone; compound e) and of pituitary adrenocorticotropic hormone on rheumatoid arthritis. Mayo Clin Proc 24:181–197

19. Hogan AC, Mcavoy CE, Dick AD, et al. (2007) Long-term efficacy and tolerance of tacrolimus for the treatment of uveitis. Ophthalmology 114:1000–1006

20. Imrie FR, Dick AD (2007) Nonsteroidal drugs for the treatment of noninfectious posterior and intermediate uveitis. Curr Opin Ophthalmol 18:212–219

21. Jabs DA, Nussenblatt RB, Rosenbaum JT (2005) Standardization of uveitis nomenclature for reporting clinical data. Results of the First International Workshop. Am J Ophthalmol 140:509–516

22. Jabs DA, Rosenbaum JT, Foster CS, et al. (2000) Guidelines for the use of immunosuppressive drugs in patients with ocular inflammatory disorders: recommendations of an expert panel. Am J Ophthalmol 130:492–513

23. Kam JC, Szefler SJ, Surs W, et al. (1993) Combination IL-2 and IL-4 reduces glucocorticoid receptor-binding affinity and T cell response to glucocorticoids. J Immunol 151:3460–3466

24. Kaspers GJL, Veerman AJP, Pieters R, et al. (1997) In vitro cellular drug resistance and prognosis in newly diagnosed childhood acute lymphoblastic leukemia. Blood 90:2723–2729

25. Langhoff E, Jakobsen BK, Ryder LP, et al. (1986) Recipient lymphocyte sensitivity to methylprednisolone affects cadaver kidney graft survival. Lancet 327:1296–1297

26. Lee RWJ, Creed TJ, Schewitz LP, et al. (2007) CD4+ CD25int T cells in inflammatory diseases refractory to treatment with glucocorticoids. J Immunol 179:7941–7948

27. Leung DY, Martin RJ, Szefler SJ, et al. (1995) Dysregulation of interleukin 4, interleukin 5, and interferon gamma gene expression in steroid-resistant asthma. J Exp Med 181:33–40

28. Leung DY, Bloom JW (2003) Update on glucocorticoid action and resistance. J Allergy Clin Immunol 111:3–22; quiz 23

29. Macphee IA, Antoni FA, Mason DW (1989) Spontaneous recovery of rats from experimental allergic encephalomyelitis is dependent on regulation of the immune system by endogenous adrenal corticosteroids. J Exp Med 169:431–445

30. Mitch WE (2000) Mechanisms accelerating muscle atrophy in catabolic diseases. Trans Am Clin Climatol Assoc 111:258–269

31. Newton R, Holden NS (2007) Separating transrepression and transactivation: a distressing divorce for the glucocorticoid receptor? Mol Pharmacol 72:799–809

32. Norman M, Hearing SD (2002) Glucocorticoid resistance—what is known? Curr Opin Pharmacol 2:723–729

33. Nussenblatt RB, Thompson DJS, Li Z, et al. (2003) Humanized anti-interleukin-2 (IL-2) receptor alpha therapy: long-term results in uveitis patients and preliminary safety and activity data for establishing parameters for subcutaneous administration. J Autoimmun 21:283–293

5

34. Nussenblatt RB, Palestine AG, Chan CC, et al. (1991) Randomized, double-masked study of cyclosporine compared to prednisolone in the treatment of endogenous uveitis. Am J Ophthalmol 112:138–146

35. Nussenblatt RB, Fortin E, Schiffman R, et al. (1999) Treatment of noninfectious intermediate and posterior uveitis with the humanized anti-tac mab: a phase I/II clinical trial. Proc Natl Acad Sci USA 96:7462–7466

36. Ohno S, Char DH, Kimura SJ, et al. (1977) Vogt–Koyanagi–Harada syndrome. Am J Ophthalmol 83:735–740

37. Perretti M (2007) Glucocorticoids in innate immunity: more transactivation than transrepression! Blood 109:852–853

38. Ramdas J, Harmon JM (1998) Glucocorticoid-induced apoptosis and regulation of NF-kappaB activity in human leukemic T cells. Endocrinology 139:3813–3821

39. Rhen T, Cidlowski JA (2005) Antiinflammatory action of glucocorticoids—new mechanisms for old drugs. N Engl J Med 353:1711–1723

40. Schaaf M, Marcel JM, Cidlowski JA (2002) Molecular mechanisms of glucocorticoid action and resistance. J Steroid Biochem Mol Biol 83:37–48

41. Schacke H, Schottelius A, Docke WD, et al. (2004) Dissociation of transactivation from transrepression by a selective glucocorticoid receptor agonist leads to separation of therapeutic effects from side effects. Proc Natl Acad Sci USA 101:227–232

42. Sliwinska-Stanczyk P, Pazdur J, Ziolkowska M, et al. (2007) The effect of methylprednisolone on proliferation of PBMCs obtained from steroid-sensitive and steroid-resistant rheumatoid arthritis patients. Scand J Rheumatol 36:167–171

43. Towler HM, Cliffe AM, Whiting PH, et al. (1989) Low dose cyclosporin A therapy in chronic posterior uveitis. Eye 3:282–287

44. Travis Sp, Farrant Jm, Ricketts C, et al. (1996) Predicting outcome in severe ulcerative colitis. Gut 38:905–910

45. Ullian ME (1999) The role of corticosteriods in the regulation of vascular tone. Cardiovasc Res 41:55–64

46. Webster JI, Tonelli L, Sternberg EM (2002) Neuroendocrine regulation of immunity. Annu Rev Immunol 20:125–163

47. Zelazowska EB, Singh A, Raybourne RB, et al. (1997) Lymphocyte subpopulation expression in women: effect of exercise and circadian rhythm. Med Sci Sports Exerc 29:467–473

Chapter 6

Multiple Sclerosis and Uveitis

6

Graeme J. Williams

Core Messages

- Most common in young adults or middle-aged Caucasians with female preponderance
- Prevalence of uveitis in patients with MS is 1.1–2.4%
- Prevalence of MS in patients with uveitis is 1–1.3%
- No temporal association between the development of MS and uveitis
- No pattern of MS that correlates with the development of uveitis
- Uveitis is generally bilateral, and may be anterior, intermediate or posterior
- Anterior uveitis may be granulomatous in up to 50% patients and posterior synaechiae may develop
- Posterior uveitis findings may include retinal vasculitis, vitritis, peripheral retinal ischaemia, retinal neovascularisation and peripheral periphlebitis
- Steroids are the mainstay of treatment
- Interferon-β appears to be effective

6.1 Introduction

Optic neuritis has a well-recognised association with multiple sclerosis (MS). Forty-five percent of patients with MS have been found to have optic atrophy at post mortem [1]. Although MS predominantly involves the optic nerves [2] and the pathways controlling eye movements [3], there also appears to be an association between MS and uveitis.

Retinal periphlebitis was first reported in association with MS in 1944 [4]. There are numerous case reports/series in the literature reporting an association between MS and uveitis [5, 6].

The association between uveitis and MS has been reported to have a significant female preponderance [7–9]. It is found most commonly in young adult or middle-aged Caucasians [7].

6.2 Association Between Multiple Sclerosis and Uveitis

The prevalence of MS-associated uveitis in previous series has varied between 0.4 and 27% [10–13]. Some of these studies are rather historic and were undertaken prior to defined diagnostic guidelines and access to magnetic resonance imaging. This may account for such a high prevalence in some series. Recent large studies have found the prevalence of uveitis in patients with MS to be 1.1–2.4% [8, 14], and the prevalence of MS in patients with uveitis to be 1–1.3% [7, 8, 15]. This is ten times the predicted prevalence of uveitis for the general population.

There appears to be no temporal association between the development of uveitis and MS [7]. The diagnosis of MS may occur before, concurrently or after the diagnosis of MS [7, 8, 16]. In one study 56% had a diagnosis of MS prior to onset of uveitis, 19% concurrently and 25% between three and nine years after their uveitis. In those patients with a diagnosis of MS prior to their presentation with uveitis, the diagnosis had been made between one and 19 years previously [7]. There is a report of a child presenting at eight years of age with bilateral intermediate uveitis who didn't develop further neurological symptoms for 13 years, when a definite diagnosis of MS was made [17]. Isolated granulomatous anterior uveitis has been described as occurring up to 22 years before the first clinical manifestations of MS [18].

There appears to be no specific pattern or duration of MS that correlates with the development of uveitis.

In one series MS was relapsing–remitting in 19 of 28 patients (67.8%), secondary progressive in eight of 28 patients (28.6%), and primary progressive in one patient [8]. These findings are consistent with previous studies [12, 19].

In general, patients with evidence of inactive MS-associated uveitis on routine examination deny previous ocular symptoms. One series of patients with MS but no ocular symptoms found 18% to have ocular vascular abnormalities consistent with uveitis [19]. All patients in that study with active uveitis had active neurological disease. It was suggested that retinal vasculitis may represent the visible correlate of concomitant active CNS demyelination, as had previously been suggested [20], and that the presence of uveitis may be a useful marker of MS disease activity [19].

There appears to be an association between MS, uveitis and autoimmune disease. However, the aetiology of MS and uveitis remain unknown. It may be that patients with both uveitis and MS, although having a similar disease to MS, are actually aetiologically distinct [8]. However, there does not appear to be any clinical or radiological distinction between patients with MS that have concomitant or an absence of uveitis [21]. It has been suggested there may be a familial association between patients with MS and relatives with autoimmune diseases, including uveitis [22]. There appears to be an association between the HLA-DR15 allele and a predisposition to MS and pars planitis [23]. The question therefore is whether the association between MS and uveitis is direct, or an increased genetic susceptibility to autoimmune disease in general, including MS, within this population [8, 24].

6.3   Clinical Findings in MS-Associated Uveitis

When uveitis is present in association with MS it is generally bilateral [6, 7, 15, 16, 20, 25, 26]. Uveitis may be anterior, intermediate or posterior. In patients with anterior uveitis, up to 50% are granulomatous in nature [6, 7, 9, 15, 16, 27, 28] (Fig. 6.1) and posterior synechiae may develop [9].

Findings of posterior uveitis in association with MS can take a number of forms, including retinal vasculitis [29] (Figs. 6.2 and 6.3) that may be occlusive, vitritis [20], peripheral retinal ischaemia and retinal neovascularisation [26], and peripheral periphlebitis [4].

Only asymptomatic peripheral periphlebitis with optic neuritis appears to have a diagnostic value for predicting the future development of MS [30]. All other findings, although associated with MS, are nonspecific and may occur in association with other disorders. Complications that occasionally arise include retinal neovascularisation, rubeosis, glaucoma, cataract and vitreous haemorrhage [31].

In one large series of patients with MS, intermediate uveitis was found in 35.7% of those affected and panuveitis in 39.3%. 14.3% of the patients had isolated anterior uveitis, 10.7% posterior uveitis and 39.3% retinal periphlebitis. 78.5% of the patients had bilateral uveitis [8].

There appears to be a very strong association between MS and pars planitis. In patients with pars planitis, the prevalence of demyelinating disease, either associated MS or optic neuritis, ranges from 11–22% depending on the study [7, 24, 25, 32]. In one series of patients with pars planitis, 14.8% went on to develop MS during follow-up [24]. One North American tertiary referral centre for uveitis found that 50% of patients with MS-associated uveitis had a pars planitis [15]. Up to 48% patients with pars planitis have been found to have demyelinating lesions on magnetic resonance brain imaging [33].

A large prospective study found the following complications in their patients with pars planitis; macular edema (47.7%), vitreous opacities (38.6%), papillitis (38.6%), vasculitis (36.4%), and cataract (20.5%) [33]. Despite these complications, good visual acuity is generally maintained; (90.9%) had a final bilateral VA better than 20/40 [33].

Up to 10% patients with retinal vasculitis go on to develop MS [29], and retinal vascular sheathing has been reported to be present in 20–36% patients with MS [11, 30, 34, 35]. It has been reported that perivascular sheathing is associated with an increased severity of progression of neurological dysfunction [11, 36]. However, opinion continues to vary with regard to the correlation between MS disease activity and retinal periphlebitis [8, 37–39]. Peripheral periphlebitis is often associated with inflammation of the pars plana/ciliary body and vitreous. Coexistent cystoid macular oedema may be present with reduced visual function [40].

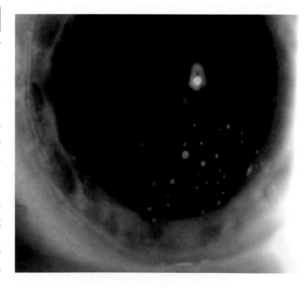

Fig. 6.1 Granulomatous anterior uveitis

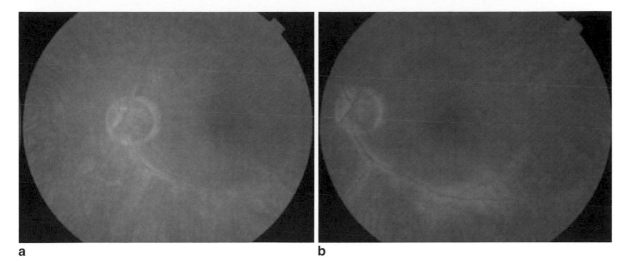

a   b

Fig. 6.2 a Late phase of fluorescence angiogram in a patient with retinal vasculitis. **b** Very late phase of fluorescence angiogram in a patient with retinal vasculitis

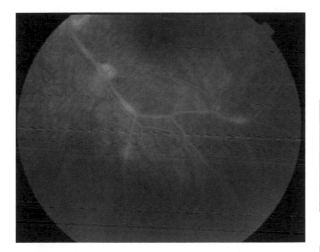

Fig. 6.3 Fluorescence angiogram showing patches of venulitis

It has previously been suggested that patients with both neurological disease and retinal vascular abnormalities may be divided into three separate groups [19]:

1. Those with a diagnosis of MS, having established neurological disease, no ocular symptoms, but for which ophthalmic examination reveals vitreous cells, peripheral venous sheathing and/or focal cuffing of the retinal veins.
2. Patients presenting with symptomatic floaters due to vitritis. Examination reveals sheathing of peripheral retinal vessels and diffuse vascular leakage demonstrated on fluorescein angiography.
3. Patients with both symptomatic ocular and neurological disease at presentation. Severe periphlebitis, retinal vein occlusion with subsequent neovascularisation

and vitreous haemorrhage. This pattern is actually rarely due to MS and occurs much more frequently in tuberculosis, sarcoidosis and systemic vasculitides. The neurological component is usually monophasic and most often consists of a spastic paresis.

Summary for the Clinician

- Only asymptomatic peripheral periphlebitis with optic neuritis appears to have a diagnostic value for predicting the future development of MS
- There is a strong association between MS and pars planitis

6.4   Histopathological Findings

One histological study involved examination of the retinas of eyes from patients with a known diagnosis of MS [34]. Eyes were obtained either at post mortem or from an eye bank. The group found histological evidence of cyclitis in 3.8% patients, choroiditis in 11.5% patients, retinal arteritis in 3.8% patients and retinal phlebitis in 20% patients. Two patterns of sheathing were identified, as previously described [35]. One suggestive of an active phlebitis showed lymphocytic infiltrate in and around the retinal veins. The second, presumably inactive venous sheathing, consisted of thickening of the vein walls, with collagen deposition. In this group, minimal cellular infiltrate was present. Interestingly, no pars planitis was reported in this group [34]. Other histopathological studies have confirmed a retinal vasculitis in association with MS [35, 36, 41, 42].

6

6.5 Experimental Models

Experimental autoimmune encephalomyelitis (EAE) has been studied in a number of animal models [43]. In the murine relapsing EAE model, a clinical picture of a relapsing–remitting form of MS develops [44, 45]. Anterior uveitis develops late in this model [46]. Interestingly, unlike the experimental autoimmune uveoretinitis model (EAU), there were no retinal changes in this EAE model [46]. Anterior uveitis has been identified as a feature of a number of EAE models in other animals, including monkey [47] and rat [48, 49]. Retinal vascular changes have been reported in some models [48, 50, 51]. It has been suggested that new antigenic determinants that may be shared between the eye and CNS are exposed to new immune cells and result in the development of uveitis [46].

The EAE model in the Lewis rat exhibits inflammatory changes in the iris, retina, optic nerve and central nervous system. The ultrastructural findings in this model suggested that the anterior uveitis was a result of vasculitis in the iris due to changes in the endothelial cells. Inflammatory cells in the form of lymphocytes and macrophages were found in the perivascular stroma of the anterior iris. Endothelial changes were also identified in the retina. In both the iris and retina, the vascular changes involved the endothelial cells taking on the appearance of high endothelial-like venules (HELV). These HELV changes were also identified in the subpial vessels in the optic nerve and in small vessels in necrotic areas in the midbrain [48].

It had previously been found that lymphocytes accumulated around small veins or venules but not around arterioles in both EAE and MS [52, 53]. HELV changes support these histopathological findings of increased perivenous lymphocytic infiltration found in the CNS and retina. It has been suggested that that these HELV changes may be the result of cytokine release from inflammatory cells due to the presence of myelin in these tissues [48]. So far there have been no reports of such HELV changes in the retina or iris of patients with MS-associated uveitis.

Summary for the Clinician

■ Antigenic determinants may be shared between the eye and the CNS

6.6 Treatment

Prolonged courses of intravenous corticosteroids have been considered a useful treatment for the management of MS-associated uveitis in patients unresponsive to oral prednisolone therapy or with concurrent active neurological disease [54]. Although predictable side effects do occur with the use of high-dose intravenous methylprednisolone, including psychological disturbance, weight gain, hypertension and hyperglycaemia, these are generally well tolerated [54–56]. Cerebral venous thrombosis has, however, been reported following the use of intravenous methylprednisolone in a patient with MS-associated uveitis [57].

Ciclosporin has previously been used effectively in the treatment of steroid-resistant MS-associated uveitis [58].

Interferon-β is accepted as having a role in the treatment of patients with MS [59, 60]. The results of the Controlled High-Risk Subjects Avonex Multiple Sclerosis Prevention Study (CHAMPS) [61] have shown a 50% reduction risk of progression to clinically definite MS in patients with optic neuritis and two or more demyelinating lesions in the brain. This has resulted in recommendations with regard to the use of interferon-β1a in patients presenting with a first episode of demyelinating optic neuritis [62]. Interferon-β appears also to be effective in the treatment of MS-associated uveitis [63]. In a group of patients with uveitis refractory to corticosteroids, there was a significant reduction in intraocular inflammation, cystoid macular oedema, and an improvement in visual acuity with interferon-β therapy [64].

The potential for tumour necrosis factor (TNF) blockers to precipitate demyelinating disease is well recognised [65]. These treatments should therefore be avoided in the treatment of identified MS-associated uveitis.

Summary for the Clinician

■ Steroids are the mainstay of treatment, though ciclosporin has been used
■ Interferon-β appears to be effective in the treatment of MS-associated uveitis
■ TNF blockers should be avoided when treating MS-associated uveitis

References

1. Rodriguez A, Calonge M, Pedroza-Seres M, Akova YA, Messmer EM, D'Amico DJ, Foster CS (1996) Referral patterns of uveitis in a tertiary eye care center. Arch Ophthalmol 114(5):593–599
2. McDonald WI, Barnes D (1992) The ocular manifestations of multiple sclerosis. I. Abnormalities of the afferent visual system. J Neurol Neurosurg Psychiatry 55:747–752
3. Barnes D, McDonald WI (1992) The ocular manifestations of multiple sclerosis. II. Abnormalities of eye movements. J Neurol Neurosurg Psychiatry 55:863–868

4. Rucker CW (1945) Sheathing of the retinal veins in multiple sclerosis. JAMA 127:970–973

5. Chebel S, Boughammoura A, Hizem Y, Frih-Ayed H (2005) Definite multiple sclerosis and uveitis: a two cases report. Eur J Neurol (12):729–731

6. Lim JI, Tessler HH, Goodwin JA (1991) Anterior granulomatous uveitis in patients with multiple sclerosis. Ophthalmol 98:142–145

7. Zein G, Berta A, Foster CS (2004) Multiple sclerosis-associated uveitis. Ocul Immunol Inflamm 12:137–142

8. Biousse V, Trichet C, Bloch-Michel E, Roullet E (1999) Multiple sclerosis associated with uveitis in two large clinic-based series. Neurology (52):179–181

9. Acar MA, Birch MK, Abbot R, Rosenthal AR (1993) Chronic granulomatous anterior uveitis associated with multiple sclerosis. Graefe's Arch Clin Exp Ophthalmol 231:166–168

10. James DG, Friedman AI, Graham E (1976) Uveitis. A series of 368 patients. Trans Ophthalmol Soc UK 96:151–157

11. Bamford CR, Ganley JP, Sibley WA, Laguna J (1978) Uveitis, perivenous sheathing and multiple sclerosis. Neurology 28:119–124

12. Breger BC, Leopold IH (1966) The incidence of uveitis in multiple sclerosis. Am J Ophthalmol 62:540–545

13. Rothova A, Buitenhuis H, Meenken C, et al. (1992) Uveitis and systemic disease. Br J Ophthalmol 76:137–141

14. Edwards LJ, Constantinescu CS (2004) A prospective study of conditions associated with multiple sclerosis in a cohort of 658 consecutive outpatients attending a multiple sclerosis clinic. Mult Scler 2004 10:575–581

15. Smith JR, Rosenbaum JT (2004) Neurological concomitants of uveitis. Br J Ophthalmol 88:1498–1499

16. Porter R (1972) Uveitis in association with multiple sclerosis. Br J Ophthalmol 58:478–481

17. Jordan JF, Walter P, Ayertey HD, Brunner R (2003) Intermediate uveitis in childhood preceding the diagnosis of multiple sclerosis: a 13-year follow-up. Am J Ophthalmol 135:885–886

18. Hanes G, Staugaitis SM, Meisler DM, Lee MS (2004) Isolated granulomatous uveitis presenting twenty-two years before multiple sclerosis. J Neuroophthalmol 24:346–347

19. Graham EM, Francis DA, Sanders MD, Rudge P (1989) Ocular inflammatory changes in established multiple sclerosis. J Neurol Neurosurg Psychiatry 52:1360–1363

20. Archambeau PL, Hollenhorst RW, Rucker CS (1965) Posterior uveitis as a manifestation of multiple sclerosis. Mayo Clin Proc 40:544–551

21. Schmidt S, Wessels L, Augustin A, Klockgether T (2001) Patients with multiple sclerosis and concomitant uveitis/periphlebitis retinae are not distinct from those without intraocular inflammation. J Neurol Sci 187:49–53

22. Heinzlef O, Alamowitch S, Sazdovitch V, Chillet P, Joutel A, Tournier-Lasserve E, Roullet E (2000) Autoimmune diseases in families of French patients with multiple sclerosis. Acta Neurol Scand 101:36–40

23. Raja SC, Jabs DA, Dunn JP, et al. (1999) Pars planitis: clinical features class II HLA associations. Ophthalmol 106:594–599

24. Malinowski SM, Pulido JS, Folk JC (1993) Long term visual outcome and complications associated with pars planitis. Ophthalmology 100:818–825

25. Chester GH, Blach RK, Cleary PE (1976) Inflammation in the region of the vitreous base: pars planitis. Trans Ophthalmol Soc UK 96:151–157

26. Vine AK (1992) Severe periphlebitis, peripheral retinal ischaemia, and preretinal neovascularization in patients with multiple sclerosis. Am J Ophthalmol 113:28–32

27. Bachman CR, Rosenthal AR, Beckingsale AB (1985) Granulomatous uveitis in neurological disease. Br J Ophthalmol 69:192–196

28. Inoue K, Numaga J, Joko S, Izumi S, Kato S, Kawashima H, Fujino Y (2001) A case of multiple sclerosis with granulomatous uveitis in Japan—use of the antilipoarabinomannan (LAM)-B test in differential diagnosis. Am J Ophthalmol 131:524–526

29. Sauders MD (1987) Retinal arteritis, retinal vasculitis and autoimmune retinal vasculitis. Eye 1:441–465

30. Lightman S, McDonald WI, Bird AC, Francis DA, Hoskins A, Batchelor JR, et al. (1987) Retinal venous sheathing in multiple sclerosis. Its significance for the pathogenesis of multiple sclerosis. Brain 110:405–414

31. Towler HA, Lightman S (2000) Symptomatic intraocular inflammation in multiple sclerosis. Clin Exp Ophthalmol 28:97–102

32. Zierhut M, Foster CS (1992) Multiple sclerosis, sarcoidosis, and other diseases in patients with pars planitis. Dev Ophthalmol 23:41–47

33. Prieto JF, Dios E, Gutierrez JM, Mayo A, Calonge M, Herreras JM (2001) Pars planitis: epidemiology, treatment, and association with multiple sclerosis. Ocul Immunol Inflamm 9:93–102

34. Kerrison JB, Flynn T, Green R (1994) Retinal pathological changes in multiple sclerosis. Retina 14:445–451

35. Arnold AC, Pepose JS, Hepler RS, Foos RY (1984) Retinal periphlebitis and retinitis in multiple sclerosis: I. Pathologic characteristics. Ophthalmol 91:255–262

36. Engell T, Hvidberg A, Uhrenholdt A (1984) Multiple sclerosis: periphlebitis retinalis and cerebrospinalis. A correlation between periphlebitis retinalis and abnormal technectium brain scintigraphy. Acta Neurol Scand 69:293–297

37. Jabs DA, Johns CJ (1986) Ocular involvement in chronic sarcoidosis. Am J Ophthalmol 102(3):297–301

38. Shah SM, Howard RS, Sarkies NJ, Graham EM (1988) Tuberculosis presenting as retinal vasculitis. J R Soc Med 81(4):232–233

39. Mochizuki M, Knwabara T, McAllister C, Nussenblatt RB, Gery I (1985) Adoptive transfer of experimental autoimmune uveoretinitis in rats. Immunopathologic mechanisms and histologic features. Invest Ophthalmol Vis Sci 26(1):1–9

40. Dick AD (1999) Immune regulation of uveoretinal inflammation. Dev Ophthalmol 30:187–202

41. Toussaint D, Perier O, Verstappen A, Bervoets S (1983) Clinicopathological study of the visual pathways, eyes, and cerebral hemispheres in 32 cases of disseminated sclerosis. J Clin Neuroophthalmol 3:211–220

42. Shaw PJ, Smith NM, Ince PG, Bates D (1987) Chronic periphlebitis retinae in multiple sclerosis. A histopathological study. J Neurol Sci 77:147–152

43. Constantinescu CS, Hilliard B, Fujioka T, Bhopale MK, Calida D, Rostami AM (1998) Pathogenesis of neuroimmunologic diseases. Experimental models. Immunol Res 17:217–227

44. Fritz RB, Chou JC-H, McFarlin DE (1983) Relapsing murine experimental allergic encephalomyelitis induced by myelin basic protein. J Immunol 130:1024–1026

45. Fritz RB, Chou JC-H, McFarlin DE (1983) Induction of experimental allergic encephalomyelitis in PL/J and (SJL/JxPL/J)F1 mice by myelin basic protein and its peptides: localization of a second encephalitogenic determinant. J Immunol 130:191–194

46. Constantinescu CS, Lavi E (2000) Anterior uveitis in murine relapsing experimental autoimmune encephalomyelitis (EAE), a mouse model of multiple sclerosis (MS). Curr Eye Res 20:71–76

47. Hayreh SS (1981) Experimental allergic encephalomyelitis. II. Retinal and other ocular manifestations. Invest Ophthalmol Vis Sci 21:270–281

48. Shikishima K, Lee WR, Behan WM, Foulds WS (1993) Uveitis and retinal vasculitis in acute experimental allergic encephalomyelitis in the Lewis rat: an ultrastructural study. Exp Eye Res 56:167–175

49. Verhagen C, Mor F, Cohen IR (1995) T cell immunity to myelin basic protein induces anterior uveitis in Lewis rats. J Neuroimmunol 53:65–71

50. von Sallmann L, Myers RE, Lerner EM, Stone SH (1967) Vaso-occlusive retinopathy in experimental allergic encephalomyelitis. Arch Ophthalmol 78:112–120

51. Hu P, Pollard J, Hunt N, Chan-Ling T (1998) Microvascular and cellular responses in the retina of rats with acute experimental allergic encephalomyelitis (EAE). Brain Pathol 8:487–498

52. Behan PO, Kies MW, Lisak RP, Sheremata W, Lamarche JB (1973) Immunologic mechanisms in experimental encephalomyelitis in nonhuman primates. Arch Neurol 29:4–9

53. Adams CWM, Poston RN, Buk SJ, Sidhu YS, Vipond H (1985) Inflammatory vasculitis in multiple sclerosis. J Neurol 69:269–283

54. Wakefield D, Jennings A, McCluskey PJ (2000) Intravenous pulse methylprednisolone in the treatment of uveitis associated with multiple sclerosis. Clin Exp Ophthalmol 28:103–106

55. Wakefield D, McCluskey PJ, Penny R (1986) Intravenous pulse methylprednisolone in severe inflammatory eye disease. Arch Ophthalmol 104:847–851

56. McCluskey PJ, Wakefield D (1987) Intravenous pulse methylprednisolone in scleritis. Arch Ophthalmol 105:793–797

57. Kadayifcilar S, Gedik S, Eldem B, Balaban H, Kansu T (2004) Panuveitis associated with multiple sclerosis complicated by cerebral venous thrombosis. Ocul Immunol Inflamm 12:153–157

58. Nussenblatt RB, Palestine AG, Chan C-C, Breen L, Caruso R (1984) Improvement of uveitis and optic nerve disease by cyclosporine in a patient with multiple sclerosis. Am J Ophthalmol 97:790–791

59. Lubin F (2005) History of modern multiple sclerosis therapy. J Neurol 252(Suppl 3):III3–III9

60. Panitch H, Goodin D, Francis G, et al. (2005) Benefits of high-dose, high-frequency interferon beta 1a in relapsing-remitting multiple sclerosis are sustained to 16 months: final comparative results of the EVIDENCE trial. J Neurol Sci 239:67–74

61. Galetta SL (2001) The controlled high risk avonex multiple sclerosis trial (CHAMPS study). J Neuroophthalmol 21:292–295

62. CHAMPS Study Group (2001) Interferon beta-1a for optic neuritis patients at high risk for multiple sclerosis. Am J Ophthalmol 132:463–471

63. Mackensen F, Max R, Becker MD (2006) Interferon therapy for ocular disease. Curr Opin Ophthalmol 17:567–573

64. Becker MD, Heligenhaus A, Hudde T, Storch-Hagenlocher B, Wildemann B, Barisani-Asenbauer T, Thimm C, Stubiger N, Fiehn C (2005) Interferon as a treatment for uveitis associated with multiple sclerosis. Br J Ophthalmol 89:1254–1257

65. Mohan N, Edwards ET, Cupps TR, et al. (2001) Demyelination occurring during anti-tumour necrosis factor alpha therapy for inflammatory arthritides. Arthritis Rheum 44:2862–2869

Chapter 7

Inflammation in Age-Related Macular Degeneration: What is the Evidence?

Heping Xu, John V. Forrester

7

Core Messages

- Immune-related gene polymorphism predisposes to age-related macular degeneration (AMD). Other environmental factors such as cigarette smoking, nutrition, and possibly chronic infection are required for the development of AMD.
- Inflammation is involved in the pathogenesis of both "dry" and "wet" types of AMD.
- Although AMD is a chronic age-related inflammatory eye disease, no "golden" serum marker that can predict AMD development or progression has been identified.
- Dysregulation of immune function in AMD mainly involves the innate immune response, including complement activation and myeloid cell dysfunction.
- In "dry" AMD, complement activation at Bruch's membrane and dysfunction of choroidal macrophage/dendritic cells may be involved in drusen formation.

- In "wet" AMD, complement activation and choroidal macrophage recruitment are involved in choroidal neovascularization (CNV).
- Various complement components and complement regulatory factors are produced locally in ocular tissues, and a local complement regulation system may exist in the eye. However, the key triggers for complement activation in AMD are not known.
- During physiological aging, a subset of retinal microglia migrates to the subretinal space and becomes activated. The activation and migration of retinal microglia are more pronounced in AMD. However, whether they are neuroprotective or neurotoxic in AMD warrants further investigation.
- Nonspecific systemic anti-inflammatory treatment has no consistent beneficial effect in AMD.
- Local low-grade inflammation rather than systemic chronic inflammation may play an important role in AMD pathogenesis.

7.1 Introduction

The concept that chronic inflammation may be associated with AMD has emerged over the last twenty years. Chronic inflammatory infiltrates (macrophages, lymphocytes and mast cells) have been demonstrated in the choroid of donor eyes with AMD [1, 2]. Analyses of drusen composition in both animal models and in patients with early-stage AMD have revealed evidence of inflammatory and immune-mediated processes, including components of the complement cascade. The resurgence of interest in this concept is largely attributed to recent genetic studies in which complement factor H (a key inhibitor of the alternative pathway of complement activation) and factor B (a key factor in the activation of the alternative pathway) gene polymorphisms have been reported to be significant predisposing factors to both early and late AMD in several independent studies (see review in [3]). Over the last few years, extensive studies have revealed more evidence supporting a possible role for local/systemic inflammation in the etiology of AMD. This chapter summarizes our current understanding of the role of inflammation in the etiology of AMD and discusses some novel ideas on how inflammations may lead to the formation of drusen or subretinal neovascularization and the apoptosis of RPE/photoreceptor cells.

7

7.2 Evidence from Clinical Studies

7.2.1 Genetic Link to Inflammation

Attempts to determine genes that might be associated with a predisposition to develop AMD began in the mid-1990s [4]. The turning point came in 2005, when three independent groups uncovered a gene on chromosome 1 that greatly increases the risk of developing AMD [5–7]. The gene encodes a protein named complement factor H (CFH) that controls the activation of the complement system through the alternative pathway. Another three tightly linked genes (PLEKHA1, LOC387715 and HTRA1) in chromosome 10q26 were later reported to be highly associated with AMD susceptibility [8–11]; however, the functions of these genes are unknown. Other genetic studies also revealed replicable, but smaller, associations of several other genes, including complement factor B (CFB) [12, 13], complement C2 [12, 13], C3 [14], IL-8 [15], CX3CR1 [16], TLR4 [17] and HLA class I and HLA class II [18] with AMD. It is important to note that all of the above genes uncovered in genetic studies are inflammation-related, indicating that inflammation may play a role in AMD development. Functional studies of the CFH gene variant with Tyr402His substitution showed a reduced ability of CFH protein to bind to C reactive protein (CRP), heparin and retinal pigment epithelial (RPE) cells [19]. The effect of this reduced binding is to cause inefficient complement regulation at the cell surface, particularly when CRP is recruited to injured sites and tissues [19]. Variations in the CFH gene may therefore predispose individuals to complement activation through the alternative pathway. Functional studies on the effects of other gene variations as risk factors for AMD development are still in the early stages of investigation. It must be kept in mind, however, that association does not equate to causation, and although a strong association between a few inflammatory genes and AMD has been discovered, it does not prove causation at this point. Other environmental factors such as cigarette smoking, nutrition, and possibly chronic infection in combination with genetic variation may warrant AMD development. Further experimental and clinical studies are necessary for a full understanding of the role of inflammation in AMD.

Summary for the Clinician

- AMD is a disease with multiple gene mutations, and many of the genes are involved in various inflammatory pathways.
- Gene mutations predispose individuals to AMD development. Aging and other environmental factors are equally important for the development of AMD.

7.2.2 Epidemiological Evidence for Inflammatory Markers in AMD

Epidemiologists have carried out several population-based studies to identify systemic inflammatory markers in different types of AMD patients. Scientists are hoping to use such makers to predict the development or progression of AMD in older populations. Although a few inflammation-related proteins have been found to be strongly associated with AMD, results to date from different groups have failed to reveal consistent findings. The lack of systemic inflammatory makers may indicate that local chronic inflammation is more important than systemically derived inflammatory cues in the development of AMD. The main inflammatory markers that have been investigated are summarized below.

7.2.2.1 C-Reactive Protein (CRP)

CRP is the prototypical acute-phase serum protein, rising rapidly in response to inflammation. It is a "golden" marker of systemic inflammation and has been shown to be an independent indicator of risk for cardiovascular and peripheral arterial disease [20, 21]. In the Age-Related Eye Disease Study (AREDS) reported by Seddon and colleagues, CRP levels were significantly associated with the presence of intermediate and advanced stages of AMD [22, 23]. In line with this observation, the Rotterdam Study found that elevated baseline levels of high-sensitivity CRP (hsCRP) were associated with the development of early and late AMD [24]. In addition, a few other studies have also revealed an association between elevated CRP serum levels and AMD [25, 26], providing further support for the hypothesis that systemic signals of inflammation may play a role in AMD.

However, results from the Beaver Dam Eye Study found no association between either the prevalence or incidence of AMD and CRP [27, 28]. Similarly, there was no association between CRP levels and AMD in the Muenster Aging and Retina Study [29], the Blue Mountains Eye Study [30] and the Cardiovascular Health Study [31]. These data, therefore, do not support the theory alleging nonspecific systemic inflammation in the etiology and natural history of AMD.

7.2.2.2 IL-6

IL-6 is primarily produced at the site of inflammation and plays a key role in the acute phase immune response. Together with its soluble receptor (sIL-6R), IL-6 also plays an important role in the transition between acute and chronic inflammation [32]. In chronic inflammation, IL-6 has a detrimental role that favors mononuclear cell accumulation at the site of injury. Increased circulating IL-6 has been observed in several inflammatory diseases, including rheumatoid arthritis, systemic lupus erythematosus and Crohn's disease. Studies on the association between serum levels of IL-6 and AMD are also inconclusive. Higher levels of IL-6 were found to be independently associated with progression of AMD in the Age-Related Eye Disease Study [21]. However, in the Beaver Dam Eye Study [28] and the Blue Mountains Eye Study [30], no significant associations were observed between IL-6 and early/late AMD.

7.2.2.3 Tumor Necrosis Factor-α (TNF-α)

TNF-α is a well-recognized inflammatory cytokine that plays important roles in various inflammatory diseases. Blocking TNF-α has been shown to have beneficial effects in a number inflammatory diseases, including rheumatoid arthritis, Crohn's disease, ankylosing spondylitis, as well as uveitis [33, 34]. Cousins et al. investigated the production of TNF-α by monocytes of AMD patients and found that monocytes from patients with CNV produced more TNF-α then controls [35]. Partially activated monocytes, defined as high TNF-α expression, may be a biomarker for identifying patients at risk of the formation of choroidal neovascularization. However, in the Beaver Dam Eye Study, TNF-α was not associated with either the prevalence or the incidence of AMD [28].

7.2.2.4 Intercellular Adhesion Molecule (ICAM)-1

The intercellular adhesion molecule (ICAM) 1 is an Ig-like cell adhesion molecule expressed by several cell types, including leukocytes and endothelial cells. ICAM-1 plays important roles in various inflammatory processes, including antigen-presenting cell (APC)–T cell antigen presentation and leukocyte recruitment. ICAM-1 is shed by the cell and detected in plasma in soluble form (sICAM-1). Increased sICAM-1 has been observed in a number of inflammatory diseases and is considered a marker for systemic chronic inflammation. In the Rotterdam study, elevated circulating levels of sICAM-1 were found preceding the development of visually significant AMD in women [26]. In the Blue Mountains Eye Study, elevated ICAM-1 was found to be marginally associated with late AMD [30]. These data support the hypothesis that inflammation may play a role in AMD.

7.2.2.5 Circulating White Blood Cell (WBC) Count

An elevated WBC count may be a marker for chronic inflammation. WBC count is a strong predictor of myocardial infarction and other coronary heart diseases [36].

Data from various cross-sectional and case–control studies have been largely inconsistent. A positive association has been observed in some studies, including the Beaver Dam Eye Study [27], the Blue Mountains Eye Study [37, 38], and the study of Blumenkranz and colleagues [39]. Higher WBC counts were found to be associated with early AMD [38], large drusen and RPE degeneration [27]. However, other studies, including some reports from the Beaver Dam Eye Study [27, 28], the Muenster Aging and Retina Study [29], the Cardiovascular Health Study [31] and the Blue Mountains Eye Study [30], have found no association between WBC count and AMD. It should be noted, however, that all of the aforementioned studies investigated the total WBC count. It might be more appropriate to investigate the association of different leukocyte subsets and AMD, as recent animal studies have shown that monocytes are actively involved in AMD pathogenesis [40, 41].

7.2.2.6 Retinal Autoantibodies

Cherepanoff and colleagues sought evidence of autoimmune inflammation in AMD by studying retinal autoantibodies [42]. The odds of having retinal autoantibodies were 4.1 times greater in early AMD patients compared to age-matched controls; however, the antibody profile was complex in terms of antigenic targets and immunoglobulin subclasses [42]. Gu and colleagues found that the omega-(2-carboxyethyl)pyrrole (CEP) protein adducts derived from the free radical-induced oxidation of docosahexaenoate (DHA) were more abundant in ocular tissues from AMD patients than normal human donors [43]. Moreover, the anti-CEP antibody was detected at 2.3 times higher levels in AMD patients than in age-matched controls [43]. Anti-CEP titers may have diagnostic utility in predicting AMD susceptibility.

7.2.2.7 Other Markers

Various studies have also looked for an association between AMD and other markers, particularly hemostatic factors such as fibrinogen, homocysteine, plasminogen activator inhibitor (PAI)-1 and von Willebrand factor. Again the results were largely inconclusive. An association was observed between the increased levels of PAI-1 and both early and late AMD in a recent report from the Blue Mountains Eye Study [30]. Amyloid A, E-selectin, and folate were investigated in the Beaver Dam Eye Study, but no association with either the prevalence or incidence of AMD was observed [28].

Evidence also suggests that chronic infection, in addition to gene mutation, may be involved in AMD development

[44]. Individuals with Y402H variants of the CFH gene and a raised anti-*C. Pneumoniae* antibody titre have an almost 12-fold greater risk of developing AMD compared to those without the CFH gene variants and a lower antibody titre [44]. In a case–control study in the USA involving serum samples from 25 AMD patients and 18 controls, an association was found between AMD and anti-*C. penumoniae* antibodies, but not other microbial antibodies [45]. The involvement of *C. pneumoniae* infection in AMD was further confirmed by a few other studies [45–47]. However, there are also some negative studies that do not support this association. Kessler and colleagues investigated 13 subretinal neovascular (SRNV) membranes from AMD patients, and they found no DNA from either *C. pneumoniae* or other pathogens by PCR, indicating that *C. pneumoniae* may not be associated with the development of SRNV membranes in exudative AMD [48]. A more recent report for the Blue Mountains Eye Study [47] also failed to detect any association between *C. pneumoniae* antibody titer and the prevalence of early or late AMD.

Summary for the Clinician

- Although a few inflammation-related proteins have been shown to be strongly associated with AMD, the results from different groups are inconsistent. Their value in predicting the development of AMD or monitoring the progression of AMD is limited.
- The lack of systemic inflammatory markers in AMD suggests that local low-grade inflammation is more likely to be involved in AMD pathogenesis.
- The higher titers of retinal autoantibodies such as anti-CEP in AMD patients suggest that autoimmunity is involved in AMD development.
- Retinal autoantibody may become a biomarker for AMD patients in the future.

7.2.3 Inflammatory Components in Drusen

Drusen are the hallmark deposits associated with early AMD. The molecular and cellular constituents of drusen have been analyzed extensively [49, 50], and distinct array of molecules, including vitronectin, amyloid A/P, Factor X, prothrombin, and in some instances immunoglobulin, HLA-DR, complement C3, C5, C5b-9, CFH, and CRP [49, 51–53], have been revealed in drusen of AMD patients. Many of these drusen-associated constituents are active participants in humoral and cellular immune responses, or are components of various inflammatory responses.

7.2.4 Evidence from Clinical Anti-inflammatory Treatment Studies

Evidence supporting the concept that AMD is a chronic inflammatory disease also comes from clinical studies in which anti-inflammatory treatments have been shown to have a beneficial effect on AMD. For instance, triamcinolone acetonide is an anti-inflammatory steroid with an angiostatic effect. Intravitreal triamcinolone injection improves visual acuity in exudative macular degeneration patients [54–56]. Anecortave acetate is another angiostatic steroid. Clinical studies have also shown that posterior juxtascleral injection of anecortave has a beneficial effect in exudative AMD patients [57]. In addition, patients on long-term anti-inflammatory treatments for other diseases appear to have a significantly lower lifetime prevalence of AMD [58], suggesting that chronic inflammation may play a role in AMD development. However, the results for the effect of nonspecific anti-inflammatory treatment on the prevalence of AMD are not consistent. An earlier Blue Mountains Eye Study indicated that administration of nonsteroidal anti-inflammatory drugs (NSAIDs) or corticosteroids does not reduce the prevalence of either early or late AMD [59].

7.3 Evidence from Experimental Studies

7.3.1 Myeloid Cells in the Pathogenesis of AMD

Over the last few years, experimental studies have significantly advanced our understanding of the pathogenesis of AMD. A number of animal models of AMD have been reported. The most significant evidence from the experimental animal studies comes from AMD mouse models with monocyte dysfunction (e.g., CCR2- or CCL2-deficient mice, CX3CR1-deficient mice and CCL2/CX3CR1 double knockout mice). Precisely how monocyte dysfunction is related to the development of AMD is not known, but it is clear from these models that myeloid-derived cells play an important role in AMD pathogenesis.

7.3.1.1 Choroidal Monocytes in the Pathogenesis of AMD

Dendritic cells and macrophages belong to the family of circulating bone marrow-derived myeloid cells. In dry AMD, macrophages and dendritic cells have been observed to insert processes into drusen or other deposits (Fig. 7.1). It has been proposed that they may

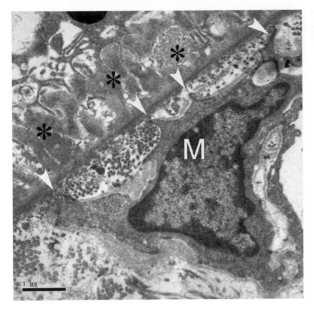

Fig. 7.1 Electron microscopy of mouse RPE/choroidal tissue shows a macrophage (M) within the Bruch's membrane, with multiple processes (*arrowheads*) towards the basement membrane of RPE. Many basal deposits (*asterisks*) are also shown

Retinal Microglial Activation During Physiological Aging

Microglia are the main immune cells in the central nerve system (CNS). Changes in microglial function reflect changes in the immune system of the CNS. In the brain, with advancing age, activated and dystrophic microglia were observed in normal physiological conditions [62, 63]. As microglia are inherently beneficial for maintaining normal brain function, deterioration of this cell population could be crucial for the development of age-related neurodegenerative disease. In the retina, microglia are normally found in the inner and outer plexiform layers, and the number and the function of retinal microglial cells are relatively stable. An earlier study observed increased numbers of rounded (activated) microglia in the aged avian retina (pigeon and quail) [64], and they were distributed mainly in regions of greatest photoreceptor loss [64]. A more recent study by Chan-Ling et al. revealed the breakdown of blood–retinal barrier, increased MHC-II in resident microglia, accompanied by activated T cells in the aged normal rat retina [65], suggesting a more primed immune system in the retina during physiological aging. We have recently shown that retinal microglia are replaced by bone marrow-derived myeloid-derived cells under normal physiological conditions. Resident retinal microglia migrate from the neuroretina to the subretinal space with age [66]. Subretinal microglia are positive for CD68 and Iba-1 and demonstrate phagocytosis activity. With age, subretinal microglia become lipofuscin-loaded autofluorescent cells [66] (Fig. 7.2). Although what causes the migration and activation of subretinal microglia is not known, such changes in the aging retina may contribute to the pathogenesis of AMD.

Microglial Activation in Age-Related Macular Degeneration

Microglial cell activation is a common immune response to ocular infections, ischemia, injury, autoimmune inflammation as well as retinal degeneration. In patients with retinitis pigmentosa, late-onset retinal degeneration and AMD, numerous activated microglia were present in the outer nuclear layer in regions of ongoing rod cell death [67]. Several studies have demonstrated early microglial cell activation in animal models of retinal degeneration, including rds (retinal degeneration slow) mice [68], the RCS (Royal College of Surgeons) rat [69] and light-induced retinal degeneration in Balb/c mice [70]. Recent studies in the mouse model of AMD (CX3CR1-deficient mice) showed a CX3CR1-dependent subretinal microglial cell accumu-

play a crucial role in the clearance of drusen and other waste materials produced by RPE cells. Dysfunction of choroidal dendritic cells or macrophages may result in the accumulation of debris or other waste materials on Bruch's membrane and ultimately the formation of drusen. This hypothesis is strongly supported by recently reported animal models of AMD, including CCR2 and CCL2 KO mice, CX3CR1 KO mice and CCL2/CX3CR1 double KO mice. CCR2 is the receptor for chemokine CCL2, whereas CX3CR1 is the cognate receptor for chemokine CX3CL1. Chemokine CCL2 and CX3CL1 are important chemoattractants for macrophages/dendritic cells. Both receptors are expressed on myeloid cells and are important for maintaining macrophage/dendritic cell functions.

For "wet" AMD, evidence for the involvement of inflammation is overwhelming. Choroidal dendritic cells/macrophages are believed to be important in the disruption of Bruch's membrane and in the formation of new subretinal blood vessels. Experiments using laser photocoagulation-induced subretinal CNV have shown that depletion of macrophages reduces the size, cellularity and vascularity of the CNV [60, 61].

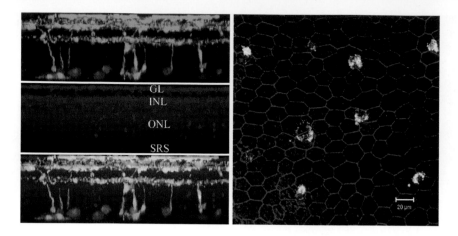

Fig. 7.2 Subretinal microglia in aged mouse retina. **a** Z-stack confocal images of retinal flatmount from a ten-month-old mouse. Retinal microglia migrate from neuroretina to subretinal space. *GL*, ganglion layer; *INL*, inner nuclear layer; *ONL*, outer nuclear layer; *SRS*, subretinal space. **b** Autofluorescent subretinal microglia in RPE flatmount from an 18-month-old mouse

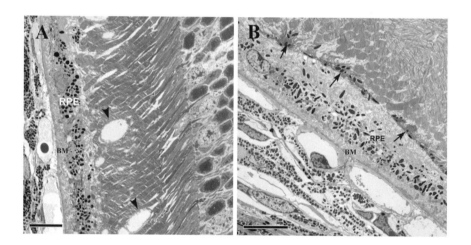

Fig. 7.3 Electron microscopy of mouse retinal/choroidal tissue. **a** TEM sample from a 24-month-old normal C57BL/6 mouse, showing a few vacuolated photoreceptor outer segments (*arrowheads*). **b** TEM sample from a 24-month-old CCL2 KO mouse, showing an area of degenerated RPE cells and accumulated subretinal microglia (*arrows*). *BM*, Bruch's membrane; *RPE*, retinal pigment epithelial cells

lation [41]. In our laboratory we have been investigating the role of retinal microglia in the pathogenesis of AMD in other AMD models (CCR2 KO mice and CCL2 KO mice). We found many more subretinal microglial cells in the aged CCR2 KO and CCL2 KO mice (Fig. 7.3) than in wild-type aged mice, and the accumulation of subretinal microglia precedes retinal degeneration.

From both human and animal studies, it is clear that microglia are one of the main immune components at the lesion site in AMD. However, what is not known to date is that whether these activated microglia are neuroprotective or neurotoxic in AMD.

Summary for the Clinician

- Choroidal dendritic cells/macrophages are important for the development of CNV.
- Microglia migrate from inner retina to subretinal space with age under normal physiological conditions; however, the function of the subretinal microglia remains to be elucidated
- In pathological conditions such as AMD, microglia accumulate in the subretinal space in the areas of RPE cell death and may be important for removing apoptotic RPE debris

7.3.2 Complement Activation in Age-Related Macular Degeneration

Genetic and immunohistochemistry studies have strongly suggested that complement activation is involved in the pathogenesis of both "dry" and "wet" AMD. A recent study in complement factor D knockout mice has shown that elimination of the alternative pathway is neuroprotective to light-induced photoreceptor damage [71]. It is therefore reasonable to suggest that in AMD, the damage to the RPE and photoreceptor cells may, at least in part, be caused directly by complement activation at the retinal/choroidal interface. Precisely how complement activation occurs in retinal tissue is not known. It is now clear that various complement components and complement regulatory factors that are usually produced in the liver are also produced locally in the eye. RPE cells have been shown to be the local source of CFH in the human eye [72]. We also found that complement factor H and factor B are both produced by RPE cells in experimental rodents [73, 74]. The production of CFB by RPE cells increases with age (Fig. 7.4). Importantly, inflammatory cytokine TNF-α positively regulates CFB production but negatively regulates CFH production in RPE cells [73, 74]. Other complement components such as C3 [75], or complement regulatory factors including membrane cofactor protein (MCP), decay-acceleration factor (DAF), membrane inhibitor of reactive lysis (CD59), and cell surface regulator of complement (Crry) have

also been detected in the retinal/choroidal tissue of normal rodent eyes [76]. These observations suggest that a local complement regulation system exists in the eye. Recently, using gene array analysis, we have observed increased inflammatory cytokine expression, including of TNF-α and others, in aged retinal tissue. It is therefore possible that increased inflammatory cytokines including TNF-α and IFN-γ, may induce CFB production but suppress CFH production. What triggers the complement activation pathway in the retina is not known. A recent study indicates that the amyloid precursor protein (APP) might serve as one of the triggers for complement activation in the aging retina, as significantly more APP is present in retinas from aged donors compared to retinas from young donors.

There is no doubt that complement activation is involved in the pathogenesis of "dry" AMD, as various complement components have been detected in drusen. Recently, experimental studies have also suggested that complement activation plays an important role in the formation of CNV [77]. Drusen complement components C3a and C5a are strong inducers of VEGF expression and may be responsible for the formation of CNV at the later stage of AMD [78]. In the laser-induced CNV model, a model for "wet" AMD, mice deficient in the complement regulatory protein CD59 developed early and severe CNV, whereas administration of recombinant soluble mouse CD59a-Fc inhibited the development of CNV [79].

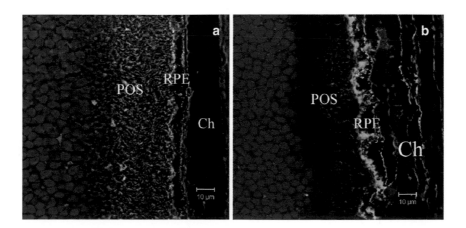

Fig. 7.4 Complement factor B (CFB) expression in mouse RPE cells. Confocal images of mouse eyes stained for CFB (*green*) and PI. **a** Sample from a three-month-old mouse; **b** sample from a 20-month-old mouse. *POS*, photoreceptor outer segments; *RPE*, retinal pigment epithelial cells; *Ch*, choroids

Summary for the Clinician

- Complement activation is involved in both "dry" and "wet" forms of AMD
- A local complement regulatory system exists at the retina/choroidal interface, and RPE cells are important cellular components of the system
- Retinal microglia may regulate RPE complement production through inflammatory cytokine/chemokine secretion

7.4 Conclusion

Evidence from clinical and experimental studies clearly indicate that AMD is an age-related chronic inflammatory disease. It largely involves the innate immune system; however, the adaptive immune system may also be involved. Polymorphisms in complement regulatory factors H and B, complement components C2, C3, chemokine receptor CX3CR1, and others predispose individuals to AMD, whereas environmental factors are essential for disease development. Although there is some evidence to show that systemic chronic inflammation might be involved in AMD, there is stronger evidence suggesting that local low-grade inflammation may be more important. The precise roles played by chronic inflammation in AMD pathogenesis are not fully understood. What triggers the inflammatory response in the retina is also unknown. Understanding how the immune response contributes to AMD pathogenesis and identifying key factors that trigger the immune response may lead to the discovery of new therapeutic approaches.

References

1. Penfold PL, Killingsworth MC, Sarks SH (1985) Senile macular degeneration: the involvement of immunocompetent cells. Graefes Arch Clin Exp Ophthalmol 223:69–76
2. Penfold PL, Liew SC, Madigan MC, Provis JM (1997) Modulation of major histocompatibility complex class II expression in retinas with age-related macular degeneration. Invest Ophthalmol Vis Sci 38:2125–2133
3. Montezuma SR, Sobrin L, Seddon JM (2007) Review of genetics in age related macular degeneration. Semin Ophthalmol 22:229–240
4. Meyers SM (1994) A twin study on age-related macular degeneration. Trans Am Ophthalmol Soc 92:775–843
5. Klein RJ, Zeiss C, Chew EY, Tsai JY, Sackler RS, Haynes C, Henning AK, Sangiovanni JP, Mane SM, Mayne ST, Bracken MB, Ferris FL, Ott J, Barnstable C, Hoh J (2005) Complement factor H polymorphism in age-related macular degeneration. Science 308:385–389
6. Edwards AO, Ritter R III, Abel KJ, Manning A, Panhuysen C, Farrer LA (2005) Complement factor H polymorphism and age-related macular degeneration. Science 308:421–424
7. Haines JL, Hauser MA, Schmidt S, Scott WK, Olson LM, Gallins P, Spencer KL, Kwan SY, Noureddine M, Gilbert JR, Schnetz-Boutaud N, Agarwal A, Postel EA, Pericak-Vance MA (2005) Complement factor H variant increases the risk of age-related macular degeneration. Science 308:419–421
8. Rivera A, Fisher SA, Fritsche LG, Keilhauer CN, Lichtner P, Meitinger T, Weber B H (2005) Hypothetical LOC387715 is a second major susceptibility gene for age-related macular degeneration, contributing independently of complement factor H to disease risk. Hum Mol Genet 14:3227–3236
9. Conley YP, Jakobsdottir J, Mah T, Weeks DE, Klein R, Kuller L, Ferrell RE, Gorin MB (2006) CFH, ELOVL4, PLEKHA1 and LOC387715 genes and susceptibility to age-related maculopathy: AREDS and CHS cohorts and meta-analyses. Hum Mol Genet 15:3206–3218
10. Dewan A, Liu M, Hartman S, Zhang SS, Liu DT, Zhao C, Tam PO, Chan WM, Lam DS, Snyder M, Barnstable C, Pang CP, Hoh J (2006) HTRA1 promoter polymorphism in wet age-related macular degeneration. Science 314(5801):989–992
11. Yang Z, Camp NJ, Sun H, Tong Z, Gibbs D, Cameron DJ, Chen H, Zhao Y, Pearson E, Li X, Chien J, Dewan A, Harmon J, Bernstein PS, Shridhar V, Zabriskie NA, Hoh J, Howes K, Zhang K (2006) A variant of the HTRA1 gene increases susceptibility to age-related macular degeneration. Science 314(5801):992–993
12. Gold B, Merriam JE, Zernant J, Hancox LS, Taiber AJ, Gehrs K, Cramer K, Neel J, Bergeron J, Barile GR, Smith RT, Hageman GS, Dean M, Allikmets R (2006) Variation in factor B (BF) and complement component 2 (C2) genes is associated with age-related macular degeneration. Nat Genet 38:458–462
13. Maller J, George S, Purcell S, Fagerness J, Altshuler D, Daly MJ, Seddon JM (2006) Common variation in three genes, including a noncoding variant in CFH, strongly influences risk of age-related macular degeneration. Nat Genet 38:1055–1059
14. Maller JB, Fagerness JA, Reynolds RC, Neale BM, Daly MJ, Seddon JM (2007) Variation in complement factor 3 is associated with risk of age-related macular degeneration. Nat Genet 39:1200–1201
15. Tsai YY, Lin JM, Wan L, Lin HJ, Tsai Y, Lee CC, Tsai CH, Tsai FJ, Tseng SH (2008) Interleukin gene polymorphisms in age-related macular degeneration. Invest Ophthalmol Vis Sci 49:693–698

16. Tuo J, Smith BC, Bojanowski CM, Meleth AD, Gery I, Csaky KG, Chew EY, Chan C (2004) The involvement of sequence variation and expression of CX3CR1 in the pathogenesis of age-related macular degeneration. FASEB J 18:1297–1299

17. Zareparsi S, Buraczynska M, Branham K E, Shah S, Eng D, Li M, Pawar H, Yashar BM, Moroi SE, Lichter PR, Petty HR, Richards JE, Abecasis GR, Elner VM, Swaroop A (2005) Toll-like receptor 4 variant D299G is associated with susceptibility to age-related macular degeneration. Hum Mol Genet 14:1449–1455

18. Goverdhan SV, Howell MW, Mullins RF, Osmond C, Hodgkins PR, Self J, Avery K, Lotery AJ (2005) Association of HLA class I and class II polymorphisms with age-related macular degeneration. Invest Ophthalmol Vis Sci 46:1726–1734

19. Skerka C, Lauer N, Weinberger AA, Keilhauer CN, Suhnel J, Smith R, Schlotzer-Schrehardt U, Fritsche L, Heinen S, Hartmann A, Weber BH, Zipfel PF (2007) Defective complement control of factor H (Y402H) and FHL-1 in age-related macular degeneration. Mol Immunol 44:3398–3406

20. Abrams J (2003) C-reactive protein, inflammation, and coronary risk: an update. Cardiol Clin 21:327–331

21. Libby P, Ridker PM (2004) Inflammation and atherosclerosis: role of C-reactive protein in risk assessment. Am J Med 116(Suppl 6A):9S–16S

22. Seddon JM, Gensler G, Milton RC, Klein ML, Rifai N (2004) Association between C-reactive protein and age-related macular degeneration. JAMA 291:704–710

23. Seddon JM, George S, Rosner B, Rifai N (2005) Progression of age-related macular degeneration: prospective assessment of C-reactive protein, interleukin 6, and other cardiovascular biomarkers. Arch Ophthalmol 123:774–782

24. Boekhoorn SS, Vingerling JR, Witteman JC, Hofman A, de Jong PT (2007) C-reactive protein level and risk of aging macula disorder: The Rotterdam Study. Arch Ophthalmol 125:1396–1401

25. Vine AK, Stader J, Branham K, Musch DC, Swaroop A (2005) Biomarkers of cardiovascular disease as risk factors for age-related macular degeneration. Ophthalmology 112:2076–2080

26. Schaumberg DA, Christen WG, Buring JE, Glynn RJ, Rifai N, Ridker PM (2007) High-sensitivity C-reactive protein, other markers of inflammation, and the incidence of macular degeneration in women. Arch Ophthalmol 125:300–305

27. Klein R, Klein BE, Marino EK, Kuller LH, Furberg C, Burke GL, Hubbard LD (2003) Early age-related maculopathy in the cardiovascular health study. Ophthalmology 110:25–33

28. Klein R, Klein BE, Knudtson MD, Wong TY, Shankar A, Tsai MY (2005) Systemic markers of inflammation, endothelial dysfunction, and age-related maculopathy. Am J Ophthalmol 140:35–44

29. Dasch B, Fuhs A, Behrens T, Meister A, Wellmann J, Fobker M, Pauleikhoff D, Hense HW (2005) Inflammatory markers in age-related maculopathy: cross-sectional analysis from the Muenster Aging and Retina Study. Arch Ophthalmol 123:1501–1506

30. Wu KH, Tan AG, Rochtchina E, Favaloro EJ, Williams A, Mitchell P, Wang JJ (2007) Circulating inflammatory markers and hemostatic factors in age-related maculopathy: a population-based case-control study. Invest Ophthalmol Vis Sci 48:1983–1988

31. McGwin G, Hall TA, Xie A, Owsley C (2005) The relation between C reactive protein and age related macular degeneration in the Cardiovascular Health Study. Br J Ophthalmol 89:1166–1170

32. Kaplanski G, Marin V, Montero-Julian F, Mantovani A, Farnarier C (2003) IL-6: a regulator of the transition from neutrophil to monocyte recruitment during inflammation. Trends Immunol 24:25–29

33. Shealy DJ, Visvanathan S (2008) Anti-TNF antibodies: lessons from the past, roadmap for the future. Handb Exp Pharmacol 181:101–129

34. Theodossiadis PG, Markomichelakis NN, Sfikakis PP (2007) Tumor necrosis factor antagonists: preliminary evidence for an emerging approach in the treatment of ocular inflammation. Retina 27:399–413

35. Cousins SW, Espinosa-Heidmann DG, Csaky KG (2004) Monocyte activation in patients with age-related macular degeneration: a biomarker of risk for choroidal neovascularization? Arch Ophthalmol 122:1013–1018

36. Hoffman M, Blum A, Baruch R, Kaplan E, Benjamin M (2004) Leukocytes and coronary heart disease. Atherosclerosis 172:1–6

37. Smith W, Mitchell P, Leeder SR, Wang JJ (1998) Plasma fibrinogen levels, other cardiovascular risk factors, and age-related maculopathy: the Blue Mountains Eye Study. Arch Ophthalmol 116:583–587

38. Shankar A, Mitchell P, Rochtchina E, Tan J, Wang JJ (2007) Association between circulating white blood cell count and long-term incidence of age-related macular degeneration: the Blue Mountains Eye Study. Am J Epidemiol 165:375–382

39. Blumenkranz MS, Russell SR, Robey MG, Kott-Blumenkranz R, Penneys N, (1986) Risk factors in age-related maculopathy complicated by choroidal neovascularization. Ophthalmology 93:552–558

40. Ambati J, Anand A, Fernandez S, Sakurai E, Lynn BC, Kuziel WA, Rollins BJ, Ambati BK (2003) An animal model of age-related macular degeneration in senescent Ccl-2- or Ccr-2-deficient mice. Nat Med 9:1390–1397

41. Combadiere C, Feumi C, Raoul W, Keller N, Rodero M, Pezard A, Lavalette S, Houssier M, Jonet L, Picard E, Debre P, Sirinyan M, Deterre P, Ferroukhi T, Cohen SY, Chauvaud D, Jeanny JC, Chemtob S, Behar-Cohen F, Sennlaub F (2007) CX3CR1-dependent subretinal microglia cell accumulation

7

is associated with cardinal features of age-related macular degeneration. J Clin Invest 117:2920–2928

42. Cherepanoff S, Mitchell P, Wang JJ, Gillies MC (2006) Retinal autoantibody profile in early age-related macular degeneration: preliminary findings from the Blue Mountains Eye Study. Clin Experiment Ophthalmol 34:590–595

43. Gu X, Meer SG, Miyagi M, Rayborn ME, Hollyfield JG, Crabb JW, Salomon RG (2003) Carboxyethylpyrrole protein adducts and autoantibodies, biomarkers for age-related macular degeneration. J Biol Chem 278:42027–42035

44. Baird PN, Robman LD, Richardson AJ, Dimitrov PN, Tikellis G, McCarty CA, Guymer RH (2008) Gene–environment interaction in progression of AMD: the CFH gene, smoking and exposure to chronic infection. Hum Mol Genet 17(9):1299–1305

45. Kalayoglu MV, Galvan C, Mahdi OS, Byrne GI, Mansour S (2003) Serological association between *Chlamydia pneumoniae* infection and age-related macular degeneration. Arch Ophthalmol 121:478–482

46. Ishida O, Oku H, Ikeda T, Nishimura M, Kawagoe K, Nakamura K (2003) Is *Chlamydia pneumoniae* infection a risk factor for age related macular degeneration? Br J Ophthalmol 87:523–524

47. Robman L, Mahdi O, McCarty C, Dimitrov P, Tikellis G, McNeil J, Byrne G, Taylor H, Guymer R (2005) Exposure to *Chlamydia pneumoniae* infection and progression of age-related macular degeneration. Am J Epidemiol 161:1013–1019

48. Kessler W, Jantos CA, Dreier J, Pavlovic S (2006) *Chlamydia pneumoniae* is not detectable in subretinal neovascular membranes in the exudative stage of age-related macular degeneration. Acta Ophthalmol Scand 84:333–337

49. Hageman GS, Mullins RF (1999) Molecular composition of drusen as related to substructural phenotype. Mol Vis 5:28

50. Anderson DH, Mullins RF, Hageman GS, Johnson LV (2002) A role for local inflammation in the formation of drusen in the aging eye. Am J Ophthalmol 134:411–431

51. Mullins RF, Russell SR, Anderson DH, Hageman GS (2000) Drusen associated with aging and age-related macular degeneration contain proteins common to extracellular deposits associated with atherosclerosis, elastosis, amyloidosis, and dense deposit disease. FASEB J 14:835–846

52. Johnson LV, Ozaki S, Staples MK, Erickson PA, Anderson DH (2000) A potential role for immune complex pathogenesis in drusen formation. Exp Eye Res 70:441–449

53. Johnson PT, Betts KE, Radeke MJ, Hageman GS, Anderson DH, Johnson LV (2006) Individuals homozygous for the age-related macular degeneration risk-conferring variant of complement factor H have elevated levels of CRP in the choroid. Proc Natl Acad Sci USA 103:17456–17461

54. Penfold PL, Gyory JF, Hunyor AB, Billson FA (1995) Exudative macular degeneration and intravitreal triamcinolone. A pilot study. Aust NZ J Ophthalmol 23:293–298

55. Jonas JB, Kreissig I, Hugger P, Sauder G, Panda-Jonas S, Degenring R (2003) Intravitreal triamcinolone acetonide for exudative age related macular degeneration. Br J Ophthalmol 87:462–468

56. Jonas JB, Kreissig I, Degenring RF (2004) Factors influencing visual acuity after intravitreal triamcinolone acetonide as treatment of exudative age related macular degeneration. Br J Ophthalmol 88:1557–1562

57. Russell SR, Hudson HL, Jerdan JA, Anecortave Acetate Clinical Study Group (2007) Anecortave acetate for the treatment of exudative age-related macular degeneration—a review of clinical outcomes. Surv Ophthalmol 52(Suppl 1):S79–S90

58. McGeer PL, Sibley J (2005) Sparing of age-related macular degeneration in rheumatoid arthritis. Neurobiol Aging 26:1199–1203

59. Wang JJ, Mitchell P, Smith W, Gillies M, Billson F, Blue Mountains Eye Study (2003) Systemic use of anti-inflammatory medications and age-related maculopathy: the Blue Mountains Eye Study. Ophthalmic Epidemiol 10:37–48

60. Espinosa-Heidmann DG, Suner IJ, Hernandez EP, Monroy D, Csaky KG, Cousins SW (2003) Macrophage depletion diminishes lesion size and severity in experimental choroidal neovascularization. Invest Ophthalmol Vis Sci 44:3586–3592

61. Sakurai E, Anand A, Ambati BK, van Rooijen N, Ambati J (2003) Macrophage depletion inhibits experimental choroidal neovascularization. Invest Ophthalmol Vis Sci 44:3578–3585

62. Streit WJ, Sammons NW, Kuhns AJ, Sparks DL (2004) Dystrophic microglia in the aging human brain. Glia 45:208–212

63. Streit WJ (2006) Microglial senescence: does the brain's immune system have an expiration date? Trends Neurosci 29:506–510

64. Kunert KS, Fitzgerald ME, Thomson L, Dorey CK (1999) Microglia increase as photoreceptors decrease in the aging avian retina. Curr Eye Res 18:440–447

65. Chan-Ling T, Hughes S, Baxter L, Rosinova E, McGregor I, Morcos Y, van Nieuwenhuyzen P, Hu P (2007) Inflammation and breakdown of the blood–retinal barrier during "physiological aging" in the rat retina: a model for CNS aging. Microcirculation 14:63–76

66. Xu H, Chen M, Manivannan A, Lois N, Forrester JV (2008) Age-dependent accumulation of lipofuscin in perivascular and subretinal microglia in experimental mice. Aging Cell 7:58–68

67. Gupta N, Brown KE, Milam AH (2003) Activated microglia in human retinitis pigmentosa, late-onset retinal degeneration, and age-related macular degeneration. Exp Eye Res 76:463–471

68. Hughes EH, Schlichtenbrede FC, Murphy CC, Sarra GM, Luthert PJ, Ali RR, Dick AD (2003) Generation of activated

sialoadhesin-positive microglia during retinal degeneration. Invest Ophthalmol Vis Sci 44:2229–2234

69. Roque RS, Imperial CJ, Caldwell RB (1996) Microglial cells invade the outer retina as photoreceptors degenerate in Royal College of Surgeons rats. Invest Ophthalmol Vis Sci 37:196–203

70. Zhang C, Shen JK, Lam TT, Zeng HY, Chiang SK, Yang F, Tso MO (2005) Activation of microglia and chemokines in light-induced retinal degeneration. Mol Vis 11:887–895

71. Rohrer B, Guo Y, Kunchithapautham K, Gilkeson GS (2007) Eliminating complement factor D reduces photoreceptor susceptibility to light-induced damage. Invest Ophthalmol Vis Sci 48:5282–5289

72. Hageman GS, Anderson DH, Johnson LV, Hancox LS, Taiber AJ, Hardisty LI, Hageman JL, Stockman HA, Borchardt JD, Gehrs KM, Smith RJH, Silvestri G, Russell SR, Klaver CCW, Barbazetto I, Chang S, Yannuzzi LA, Barile GR, Merriam JC, Smith RT, Olsh AK, Bergeron J, Zernant J, Merriam JE, Gold B, Dean M, Allikmets R (2005) From the cover: a common haplotype in the complement regulatory gene factor H (HF1/CFH) predisposes individuals to age-related macular degeneration. Proc Natl Acad Sci USA 102:7227–7232

73. Chen M, Forrester JV, Xu H (2007) Synthesis of complement factor H by retinal pigment epithelial cells is down-regulated by oxidized photoreceptor outer segments. Exp Eye Res 84:635–645

74. Chen M, Robertson M, Forrester JV, Xu H (2007) Complement factor B in retinal pigment epithelial cell is up-regulated by inflammatory cytokine TNF-alpha and IFN-gamma. Mol Immunol 44:3937

75. Coffey PJ, Gias C, McDermott CJ, Lundh P, Pickering MC, Sethi C, Bird A, Fitzke FW, Maass A, Chen LL, Holder GE, Luthert PJ, Salt TE, Moss SE, Greenwood J (2007) Complement factor H deficiency in aged mice causes retinal abnormalities and visual dysfunction. Proc Natl Acad Sci USA 104:16651–16656

76. Sohn JH, Kaplan HJ, Suk HJ, Bora PS, Bora NS (2000) Chronic low level complement activation within the eye is controlled by intraocular complement regulatory proteins. Invest Ophthalmol Vis Sci 41:3492–3502

77. Bora PS, Sohn JH, Cruz JM, Jha P, Nishihori H, Wang Y, Kaliappan S, Kaplan H J, Bora NS (2005) Role of complement and complement membrane attack complex in laser-induced choroidal neovascularization. J Immunol 174:491–497

78. Nozaki M, Raisler BJ, Sakurai E, Sarma JV, Barnum SR, Lambris JD, Chen Y, Zhang K, Ambati BK, Baffi JZ, Ambati J (2006) Drusen complement components C3a and C5a promote choroidal neovascularization. Proc Natl Acad Sci USA 103:2328–2333

79. Bora NS, Kaliappan S, Jha P, Xu Q, Sivasankar B, Harris CL, Morgan BP, Bora PS (2007) CD59, a complement regulatory protein, controls choroidal neovascularization in a mouse model of wet-type age-related macular degeneration. J Immunol 178:1783–1790

Age-Related Macular Degeneration: Immunological Factors in the Pathogenesis and Therapeutic Consequences

8

Aize Kijlstra, Ellen C. La Heij, Fleur Goezinne, Fred Hendrikse

Core Messages

- The presence of macrophages in the macular lesions of AMD patients in combination with the discovery of deposits of proteins from the complement pathway suggests that chronic low-grade inflammation plays a role in the pathogenesis of AMD.
- Activation of the complement pathway by drusen or lipofuscin fragments may form the initial triggers that activate RPE cells to release chemotactic and angiogenic cytokines followed by an influx of proinflammatory macrophages, finally leading to choroidal neovascularization.
- Photo-oxidation may lead to the formation of neo-antigens on retinal proteins. These neo-antigens may lead to the formation of autoantibodies, resulting in local immune complex formation, a further build-up of subretinal drusen, complement activation and influx of macrophages. A mouse model employing this concept has been developed and may provide a model for dry AMD.
- Two macrophage subpopulations have been identified, and each may play a different role in the aging outer retina. The so-called M1 macrophage is a proangiogenic macrophage that is stimulated via IL-10. The M2 macrophage is

a benign macrophage involved in the scavenging of cell debris. The local environment of the aging retina with regards to IL-10 release and the balance between M1 and M2 macrophages may dictate the outcome of macular lesions.

- The association of certain genetic polymorphisms of the complement protein factor H (CFH) supports the role of complement activation in AMD. CFH is thought to influence the degree of complement activation induced by drusen or photoactivation products in the outer retina.
- The intravitreal administration of humanized monoclonal antibodies against VEGF has revolutionized the treatment of wet AMD.
- Up to now there has been no treatment option for patients with the dry form of AMD. Prevention by employing a diet rich in nutrients with antioxidant or anti-inflammatory properties is currently being investigated. Macular surgery is technically difficult and has met with limited success in selected patients. Procedures include full graft translocation (RPE, Bruch's membrane and choroid) or transplantation of autologous rejuvenated RPE sheets.

8.1 Introduction

In this review we aim to highlight recent evidence implicating inflammation as a mechanism in the pathogenesis of age-related macular degeneration (AMD), and we will put forward the possible preventive and therapeutic actions that may be taken. AMD is currently considered to be the most important cause of blindness in individuals over 55 years of age in the developed world, and in view of rising life expectancy the problem is expected to increase dramatically over the coming decades unless effective preventive or therapeutic measures are developed.

A large number of potential risk factors have been identified for AMD, but the strongest associations have been observed for age and smoking [55]. In recent years a number of genetic factors involving inflammatory pathways have been discovered that also predispose individuals to acquiring AMD.

AMD is generally divided into two major forms: neovascular or exudative (wet) AMD and atrophic (dry) AMD (Fig. 8.1). Approximately 80% of the patients with wet AMD will become legally blind, as compared to 20% of eyes with dry AMD. The prevalence of dry AMD is five times higher than that of wet

8

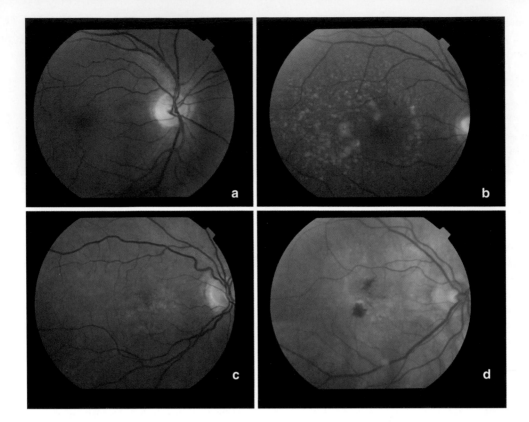

Fig. 8.1 Four pictures of the macula of the right eye. **a** A normal fundus, with a normal fovea in the center (**b**). An eye showing early age-related macular degeneration with large confluent drusen. **c** Example of an eye with dry age-related macular degeneration. **d** This panel shows the development of wet age-related macular degeneration with a subfoveal hemorrhage surrounded by RPE detachment

AMD. In the exudative form, choroidal neovascularization (CNV) finally resulting in a disciform macular scar is the cause of severe visual loss. The exudative form of AMD may be further subdivided into classic, occult or mixed-type CNV, depending on the pattern on fluorescein angiograms.

Evidence has been accumulating that immunological factors including inflammation may play an important role in the pathogenesis of AMD [32, 74]. Various as-yet unidentified triggers may initiate these immune events, and the identification of these factors may lead to new therapeutic or even preventive approaches.

8.2   Inflammatory Cells in the Choroid and Retina in AMD

A number of studies have shown the presence of inflammatory cells in the posterior segment of eyes from AMD patients [74, 82]. The presence of den-

dritic cell processes in drusen has been shown using immunofluorescence microscopy of human retinas by employing immunoreagents specific for HLA-DR and leukocytes (CD68) [32]. The choroid is known to contain a dense network of MHC class II positive dendritic cells [12, 24], but further (ultrastructural) confirmation is needed to prove that cellular processes of these cells do indeed extend through Bruch's membrane into the drusen.

Alteration of the physiology of RPE cells (degeneration, hypoxia, uptake of drusen) may potentially lead to the release of a large number of cytokines such as VEGF, MCP-1, IL-6 and IL-8 [37]. Of interest is the observation that cytokine secretion by RPE cells occurs in a polarized fashion towards the choroid [38]. Some of these cytokines induce the expression of cell adhesion molecules on vascular endothelium [76], which in combination with locally released chemokines (IL-8 or MCP-1) may lead to the influx of inflammatory leukocytes. These cells subsequently lead to a disruption of Bruch's membrane, allowing new vessels to enter the subretinal space. This scheme of events has been developed based on the outcome of recent findings using the mouse laser photocoagulation model for choroidal neovascularization (CNV).

Depletion of macrophages by clodronate-containing liposomes reduced the size, cellularity, and vascularity of the CNV lesions in this model, implicating the importance of these cells in the development of CNV [22]. The current paradigm, that macrophage infiltration promotes neovascularization in the experimental CNV model, has however been challenged by recent studies using various genetically engineered strains of knockout mice. AMD has for instance been shown to occur naturally in aged mice that have an impaired deficiency in the recruitment of macrophages (Ccl2(–/–) or Ccr2(–/–) mice) [1]. Ferguson and his group recently showed that IL-10(–/–) mice have significantly reduced CNV with increased macrophage infiltrates when compared to wild-type [4]. They also showed that prevention of macrophage entry into the eye promoted neovascularization, while local injection of macrophages inhibited CNV.

This paradigm shift can be explained as follows. Macrophages may play a role by helping RPE cells to scavenge debris. In the event that macrophage recruitment diminishes, this may lead to the accumulation of debris, leading to the recruitment of inflammatory macrophages. Macrophages have recently been subdivided into so-called M1 and M2 macrophages, of which the former is an inflammatory type of macrophage and the latter is involved in debris scavenging [28]. Decreased functioning of M2 macrophages and increased activity of M1 macrophages may both lead to AMD.

Recent studies have shown that senescence influences the outcome of CNV in the laser photocoagulation model in mice, which was attributed to an effect of age on macrophage function [53]. These authors provided evidence that IL-10 plays a key role in controlling angiogenesis. Aging was associated with increased IL-10 expression in the retinal microenvironment, which in turn triggered macrophages to become proangiogenic.

Apart from the role of macrophages recruited via the choroidal vasculature, it has also been proposed that retinal microglia may play an important role in the pathogenesis of AMD [11, 30]. The relative roles of retinal microglia vs. macrophages recruited via the choroid are not yet clear and deserve further attention.

Summary for the Clinician

- AMD has an inflammatory component in which the macrophage is the main inflammatory cell type.
- Alterations in Bruch's membrane and the presence of drusen are stimuli for RPE cells to produce chemotactic cytokines. These cytokines attract macrophages.
- M2-type macrophages are considered benign debris-scavenging cells.
- M1-type macrophages are an inflammatory type of cell that play an important role in neovascularization.
- AMD is probably the result of an altered balance between M1 and M2 macrophages in the macula.

8.3 Infectious Pathogens and AMD

Chronic infections may play a role in vascular abnormalities such as atherosclerosis [21]. Since AMD and atherosclerosis share a variety of risk factors, a number of groups have addressed the role of infectious microorganisms in the pathogenesis of AMD. Most of the interest has been focused on the role of *Chlamydia pneumoniae*. Although early studies reported an association between *Chlamydia pneumoniae* and AMD [40, 51], larger studies were not able to confirm these findings [79]. In a subsequent study, the presence of *Chlamydia pneumoniae* was established by immunohistochemistry in four out of nine CNV membranes obtained from AMD patients, as compared to none of the nine age-matched controls without AMD [50]. These authors were also able to demonstrate *Chlamydia* DNA in two out of the nine CNV membranes tested. These findings were not, however, confirmed by others [54]. If bacterial infections play a role in the pathogenesis of AMD, antibiotics may offer a means of therapy. However, the current understanding of the role of bacteria in the pathogenesis of AMD does not yet support this type of intervention.

Cytomegalovirus has also been implicated in the pathogenesis of CMV, but these findings have also not been confirmed in larger studies yet [64]. The observation that elevated white blood cell counts were shown to be associated with early AMD supports a role for systemic inflammation in the pathogenesis of AMD [83]. This is also in line with the observation of high levels of circulating acute-phase reactants in AMD, such as CRP [8].

8

Summary for the Clinician

- A role for infectious pathogens in the pathogenesis of AMD has been investigated but has not yet been proven.

8.4   Role of Autoimmunity in AMD

Autoimmunity has been considered to be one of the mechanisms that causes AMD [74]. Modern techniques using immunoblotting have shown that the retinal antibody pattern is different in AMD compared to controls [13, 43, 73]. A longitudinal follow-up of patients did not, however, reveal an association between baseline autoantibodies and the development of advanced AMD over a ten-year period [13].

A new development is a possible role for antibodies directed against modified proteins in the retina. Oxidative damage is thought to play an important role in the pathogenesis of AMD [5]. With its high levels of oxygen and various polyunsaturated fatty acids, the retina is a site that is prone to oxidative damage of proteins. Oxidative modification of retinal proteins may lead to the development of novel antigenic sites on these proteins that, in combination with an antibody response directed at these neo-antigens, may lead to local immune deposit formation. An example includes the free radical-induced oxidation of docosahexaenoate (DHA)-containing lipids, which in turn generates omega-(2-carboxyethyl)pyrrole (CEP) protein adducts. The group of Crabb has recently investigated the role of CEP protein adducts in AMD [29]. CEP is more abundant in ocular tissues from AMD patients than in normal human donors. A higher level of CEP-containing antigen was found in AMD human plasma than in age-matched controls, and sera from AMD patients had higher mean titers of anti-CEP antibody than controls. To date the role of autoimmunity against CEP in AMD has not been confirmed by other groups.

Immunization of mice with a CEP adduct of albumin results in the appearance of CEP antibodies in these animals [36]. These antibodies are able to activate the complement system in Bruch's membrane. In this animal model, drusen are formed below the RPE cell layer, and RPE lesions are observed that resemble those seen in patients with the dry form of AMD.

The fact that immunoglobulin deposits are not readily observed in the retinas of AMD eyes argues against a role for autoantibodies in AMD. Alternatively, it is possible that autoantibody formation against modified proteins is not a causative factor in AMD, but that it represents a secondary response to retinal damage. Recent observations point to a possible direct role for modified proteins in the induction of neovascularization ([19].

Summary for the Clinician

- Retinal autoantibody patterns in AMD patients are different from those in controls.
- Oxidative damage of proteins in the retina may lead to the formation of neo-antigens. An autoimmune response against retinal neo-antigens may play a role in the pathogenesis of AMD but has not yet been definitely proven.
- A mouse model of dry AMD has been developed by immunizing mice with a CEP adduct of albumin.
- The autoimmune response found in AMD may not be a causal relationship but rather a secondary phenomenon in response to retinal damage.

8.5   Drusen as Triggers of Complement Activation in AMD

Drusen are considered important risk factors in the development of AMD and can be readily observed by fundoscopic examination of the macular area [55]. They are characterized as extracellular deposits situated between the RPE cell layer and Bruch's membrane. The exact origin of drusen is not precisely known, but evidence is accumulating that their initial formation is caused by the deposition of undigested constituents derived from RPE cells. These deposits may subsequently induce an inflammatory event, leading to further depositions [2]. In combination with the recent finding of an association of AMD with genes of the complement system, this has led to a paradigm shift in relation to the role of drusen in the pathogenesis of AMD [31].

The complement system can be activated by at least three pathways: the classical pathway, the lectin pathway and the alternative pathway [68]. The classical pathway is activated through the binding of the complement system protein C1q to antigen–antibody complexes, pentraxins or apoptotic cells. The pentraxins include C-reactive protein (CRP) and serum amyloid P (SAP) component. The lectin pathway is initiated by microbial saccharides via the mannose-binding lectin (MBL). The alternative pathway can be activated after the spontaneous hydrolysis of native complement system protein C3 and requires stabilization of the activated components on suitable substrates. Activation of complement leads to the proteolytic cleavage of C4 and C3 and the formation of a covalent linkage between C4b and C3b and the activating structures. The three mentioned pathways all lead to C3 activation followed by the formation of the membrane attack complex (C5b–9).

The finding of an association of certain polymorphisms of the complement factor H (CFH) gene cluster with AMD has turned the focus onto the activation and control of the alternative pathway of complement. Central to this pathway is the alternative pathway C3 convertase, which is a complex formed by the proteins C3b and Bb. The C3bBb complex degrades native C3 and leads to further C3b deposition. The activity of the C3bBb complex is downregulated in two ways. First of all there are factors that dissociate Bb from the complex, leaving a naked C3b which is devoid of enzymatic activity but is capable of re-associating with Bb. A second process involves further cleavage of the naked C3b to C3bi, which is not able to re-associate with Bb, thereby irreversibly inactivating the C3 convertase activity. The plasma protein CFH can bind C3b and plays an important role in both processes, thereby playing a crucial role in the regulation of the enzymatic activity of the alternative pathway C3 convertase. A second biological property of CFH resides in the fact that it can bind to negatively charged surfaces such as acellular material or bacterial pathogens. The activation of the alternative complement pathway is controlled through the binding of CFH to such substances. CFH also has a binding site for CRP.

The first observation showing deposits of complement activation products in the retinas of AMD patients (Fig. 8.2) was reported by van der Schaft in 1993 [87]. These findings were confirmed eight years later by Johnson et al. [45].

Drusen are considered to contain complement proteins, but the triggers for complement activation at these sites are still unclear. Immunolabeling of AMD eyes for immune complex constituents (IgG and complement) have not always been consistent concerning the localization of IgG in the drusen [46, 69, 87], suggesting that complement activation did not occur via the classical complement pathway. Drusen have been shown to contain amyloid oligomers [60], and these deposits may be involved in the activation of the complement cascade [3, 16, 44]. Photo-oxidation of bis-retinoid pigments such as A2E that accumulate as lipofuscin in retinal pigment epithelial (RPE) cells has also been shown to activate the complement system [91]. Lipofuscin resides within the RPE cell, but photo-oxidation may lead to the release of small photo-oxidation products into the subretinal space, which may result in extracellular complement activation. Invading pathogens [26] but also CRP [8] have been considered to play a role in AMD pathogenesis, and both are also capable of activating the complement system.

Immunohistochemical studies have shown the presence of complement regulatory proteins such as vitronectin, clusterin, CR1 and CD46 (membrane cofactor protein) associated with the drusen, providing further support for a role of the complement system in the process of drusen formation (Fig. 8.3) [32]. Besides controlling complement activation, CD46 may also play an important role in the adhesion of RPE cells to the underlying Bruch's membrane [63, 88].

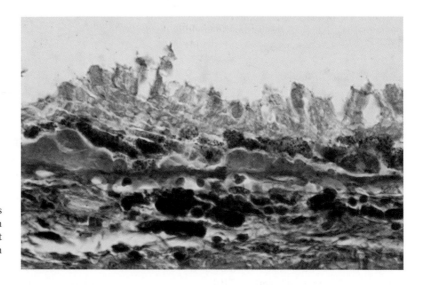

Fig. 8.2 Immunohistochemical analysis of complement component C3 deposition in a retinal section of an AMD patient with hard drusen (courtesy of Dr. T.L. van der Schaft)

8

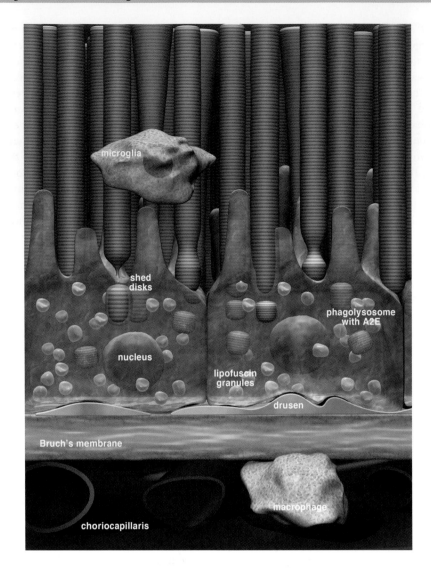

Fig. 8.3 Schematic representation of a retina from an AMD patient. Shed disks from the photoreceptors (*rods and cones*) are phagocytosed and digested by the RPE cells. Undigested material remains inside the cell as lipofuscin granules and outside the cell as drusen. The drusen contain complement activation products such as C3 and CD46 (membrane cofactor protein). Macrophages and microglia are attracted to the site to help eliminate the debris

Complement activation is associated with the generation of potent inflammatory mediators such as the complement split products C3a and C5a. RPE cells have a receptor for C5a, and stimulation of the receptor following binding to its ligand leads to mRNA synthesis of a variety of inflammatory cytokines, such as IL-1, IL-6, MCP-1 and IL-8 (Fig. 8.4) [25]. Both C3a and C5a have been shown to induce VEGF and to promote choroidal neovascularization, implicating drusen as a starting point in the pathogenesis of "wet" AMD [71].

8.6 Genetic Factors Related to Inflammation and AMD

The field of genetics in AMD was revolutionized with the discovery of an association between AMD and the complement pathway genes such as complement factor H (CFH), complement component 2 (C2) and the complement factor B (FB) [20, 27, 31, 33, 56]. A single copy of the risk-associated haplotype increased the risk of AMD approximately 2–4-fold, whereas homozygous

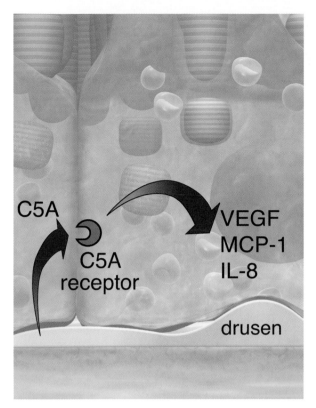

C5A

C5A
receptor

VEGF
MCP-1
IL-8

drusen

Fig. 8.4 Schematic representation of complement activation by drusen and the appearance of the complement activation product C5a. C5a can interact with its receptor on RPE cells, leading to the release of various chemotactic cytokines

individuals had a 5–7-fold increased risk. The CFH gene cluster encodes five genes, which are all expressed. To date, five CFH haplotypes have been identified, of which three predispose to AMD and two are protective. The odds ratios of the three CFH haplotypes associated with increased risk vary between 2.8 and 4.2 as compared to the protective haplotype [39]. A polymorphism in the LOC387715/HTRA1 gene region shows a much higher risk of AMD. The proteins involved are not yet clear, although HTRA1 is known to encode a serine protease. Of the four haplotypes identified in this region, one confers very high risk to AMD whereby homozygotes of haplotype 2 had a thirty times higher risk of developing AMD. Smoking status markedly worsens development of AMD in genetically susceptible persons, and a recent model has calculated that 15% of individuals belonging to these high-risk groups will eventually develop AMD [39].

The molecular basis for the roles of certain CFH polymorphisms in the pathogenesis of AMD comes from findings where it was shown that the protective variant has a higher affinity for polyanionic sites and would therefore be more efficient at controlling complement activation than the other variants [35].

No association between AMD and other genetic factors related to inflammation such as TLR4, CCL2, and CCR2 was found in preliminary studies [17].

Summary for the Clinician

- A genetic association of AMD with complement gene polymorphisms has now been shown for the complement components factor C2, factor B and complement factor H (CFH).
- The observed associations add to the proposed role of complement in the pathogenesis of AMD, whereby certain genes may lead to a disturbed regulation of complement activation.

8.7 Anti-inflammatory Effects of Nutritional Factors

Nutrition has been shown to affect the development of AMD, and further insights into consumer behavior could play an important role in the prevention of AMD. The evidence showing that supplementation with antioxidants and minerals (15 mg of beta-carotene, 500 mg of vitamin C, 400 IU of vitamin E and 80 mg zinc plus 2 mg copper) could halt the progression of AMD is mainly derived from the results of the Age-Related Eye Disease Study (AREDS) [52].

Summary for the Clinician

- Drusen are considered to be undigested cell debris material that is exocytosed by RPE cells and builds up on the inner side of Bruch's membrane.
- Drusen have been shown to contain protein fragments of the complement system.
- The complement system is a cascade of proteins that plays an important role in the battle against invading microorganisms. There are three pathways that lead to complement activation: the classical pathway, the alternative pathway, and the mannose-binding lectin pathway.
- Drusen and other substances in the vicinity of the RPE cell, such as photo-oxidized lipofuscin fragments, can lead to complement activation with subsequent deposition of the activation products such as complement factor C3 within drusen.
- Soluble complement activation products such as C5a can stimulate RPE cells to produce cytokines as VEGF, thereby initiating neovascularization.

8

The macular pigments lutein and zeaxanthin are considered to play an important role in the pathogenesis of AMD. Both observational and interventional studies indicate that these nutrients may be protective in the development of AMD [65, 77]. These pigments can prevent photo-oxidation via two mechanisms, one of which is passive while the other is an active function. First of all, they passively filter blue light and may thus prevent photo-oxidation of lipids and proteins in the retina. Both pigments are antioxidants since they can actively scavenge light-induced free oxygen radicals. Recently it was shown that lutein can inhibit the development of endotoxin-induced uveitis in rats, adding a third protective function to the macular xanthophylls [42]. The anti-inflammatory effect of lutein was comparable to that of dexamethasone. Lutein administration in rats undergoing EIU led to decreased aqueous humor levels of nitric oxide, TNF, IL-6, MCP-1, MIP-2 and PGE2 compared to controls. Lutein suppressed the activation of NF-κB in the uvea as well as the expression of iNOS and COX-2. The same group recently showed that lutein could also inhibit CNV in a laser-induced model in mice [41].

Additional evidence implicating macular pigments in AMD comes from studies where it was shown that smokers have much lower levels of macular pigments than nonsmokers [34]. Smoking is the most important environmental risk factor for AMD, and it is possible that this effect is partially mediated via low levels of macular pigment.

Other nutritional factors that may exert anti-inflammatory effects in the retina include omega-3 fatty acids [81]. Observational studies have shown that a diet rich in omega-3 fatty acids (present in fish for instance) is associated with a decreased risk of AMD [14].

In view of the current nutritional data, the National Eye Institute has developed the AREDS2 study, which has been devised to determine whether oral supplementation with lutein and zeaxanthin or omega-3 long-chain polyunsaturated fatty acids will decrease the risk of progression to advanced AMD. The study started enrolling patients in the fall of 2006. One-quarter of the patients will be assigned the placebo, another quarter to lutein and zeaxanthin, another quarter to omega-3 fatty acids, while the final quarter are assigned to the combination of the two. The fact that such a large study has been planned is an indication that the investigators have found sufficient compelling evidence for a possible major role of these nutritional factors in the prevention of AMD.

Summary for the Clinician

- Nutritional factors may influence the composition of the retina. Important nutritional factors include the macular pigments, lutein and zeaxanthin and the omega-3 fatty acids.
- The macular pigments have been shown to have anti-oxidant properties. They can prevent oxidation by passively filtering blue light and by actively scavenging free radicals.
- Lutein was recently shown to have anti-inflammatory properties.
- Omega-3 fatty acids are considered to provide an anti-inflammatory environment in the outer retina.

8.8 Anti-inflammatory Drugs and AMD

Evidence is now accumulating that inflammatory events may play a role in AMD. This would implicate a possible beneficial effect of either local or systemic treatment with anti-inflammatory drugs. Early studies did not support this hypothesis, since no association could be found between the use of systemic anti-inflammatory drugs (NSAIDs or corticosteroids) and either the cross-sectional prevalence or longitudinal incidence of ARM in the population-based cohort of the Blue Mountains Eye study [89]. However, later studies showed that local treatment may be beneficial, especially if anti-inflammatory drugs are selected with angiostatic activity.

8.8.1 Angiostatic Steroids

Triamcinolone is a promising drug with both anti-inflammatory and angiostatic effects. In vitro and experimental studies showed that it was able to inhibit choroidal neovascularization [15, 90]. The use of intravitreal triamcinolone for AMD was first described in a number of uncontrolled studies [48]. Side effects of intraocular triamcinolone include an elevated intraocular pressure, cataract formation, postoperative endophthalmitis, and rhegmatogenous retinal detachments [47, 85]. Randomized placebo-controlled studies with a one-year follow-up however showed that intravitreal triamcinolone was not beneficial for the treatment of minimally classic or occult CNV due to AMD in terms of visual acuity, contrast sensitivity, and central macular volume, and was associated with results similar to those associated with intravitreal injection of dexamethasone, which was used as placebo [59].

Anecortave acetate is another angiostatic steroid. It blocks blood vessel growth by inhibiting proteases that are necessary for vascular endothelial cell migration [75]. As compared to triamcinolone, anecortave acetate does not show the classical ocular corticosteroid side effects, such as high intraocular pressure or accelerated cataract formation. Recently performed randomized clinical trials were not able to confirm the initial positive results with this drug [18]. Further clinical studies to compare the role of angiostatic steroids in combination with verteporfin photodynamic therapy (Visudyne® PDT) are now underway [10].

Summary for the Clinician

- No association could be found between the use of systemic anti-inflammatory drugs (NSAIDs or corticosteroids) and prevalence of AMD
- Experimental studies indicated that angiostatic steroids such as triamcinolone or anecortave acetate could inhibit choroidal neovascularization
- Randomized clinical trials with angiostatic drugs showed that the clinical results in wet AMD patients were comparable to those obtained with photodynamic therapy
- Future treatments are aimed at combining photodynamic therapy with angiostatic steroid therapy

8.8.2 Antiangiogenic Therapy in AMD

The wet form of AMD is due to the formation of new choroidal vessels (neovascularization) or CNV in the central retina or macula. Treatment of wet AMD is aimed at destroying these new vessels. Until ten years ago, conventional laser photocoagulation to destroy the vessels was the only available therapy that could slow down visual loss in eyes with CNV. However, as well as attacking the CNV, conventional laser treatment destroys photoreceptor cells and other neuronal retinal cells. The introduction of photosensitizers such as verteporfin has led to a more selective targeting of the neovasculature. Large randomized clinical trials have now proven its effect, and photodynamic therapy (PDT) using verteporfin has largely replaced conventional laser therapy in eyes with subfoveal CNV [9].

Further refinement of the antiangiogenic therapy is directed at VEGF. VEGF is a key cytokine controlling angiogenesis and has been implicated in neovascularization during wet AMD [23]. The biological actions of VEGF are mediated via two receptors, VEGFR-1 and VEGFR-2. VEGF expression was shown to be increased in the maculae of human eye bank eyes with AMD [57], and also in surgically removed human CNV membranes [58]. A small VEGF-inhibiting oligonucleotide (pegaptanib or Macugen) was shown to inhibit choroidal neovascularization and was the first anti-VEGF drug that was approved to treat AMD patients [70]. A major breakthrough in the treatment of choroidal neovascularization came with the introduction of recombinant humanized monoclonal antibodies against VEGF (Avastin and Lucentis) [80, 84].

CNV can also be selectively targeted via chimeric fusion proteins composed of factor VII, the natural ligand for tissue factor, conjugated to the Fc domain of an IgG1 immunoglobulin. Factor VII binds with high affinity to tissue factor, which is selectively expressed on neovascular endothelial cells but not in the normal retinal or choroidal vessels. After the binding of the chimeric antibody, the endothelial cells are cytolysed via an Fc domain-mediated action involving natural killer cells and activation of the complement system. Treatment of animals (pigs) with this fusion protein prevented the formation of laser-induced choroidal neovascularization [86].

Other targets could include pigment epithelium-derived factor (PEDF), which is one of the most potent antiangiogenic factors known to be present in the posterior segment of the eye. Intravitreal administration of an adenovirus vector expressing PEDF was shown to be effective in the inhibition of neovascularization in a murine model of CNV [67].

8.8.3 Immunotherapy for AMD

Nussenblatt considers AMD a disease in which a change has occurred in the ocular immune microenvironment [72]. Instead of a microenvironment that is characterized by a downregulation of the immune response, it has changed into an environment with an upregulated immune response, leading to systemic recruitment of immune cells. According to this hypothesis, various systemic immunotherapies using antibodies against T cells, TNF (infliximab) or IL-2 receptor (daclizumab) or other immunosuppressive agents could be envisioned.

Given the importance of complement in the pathogenesis of AMD, the role of pharmacological intervention

8

in this pathway needs to be explored. Various drugs targeting the complement system are now being tested in clinical trials, including synthetic analogs of C5a [66, 78]. The FDA has recently approved eculizumab, an antibody directed against C5, for the treatment of paroxysmal nocturnal hemoglobinuria, but the indications are not limited to this disease [78]. Targeting C5, via intravitreal eculizumab administration, may be relevant in AMD since RPE cells have a receptor for C5a and can be triggered to produce cytokines following activation of this receptor [25]. Recently, a small peptide drug has been developed that is able to prevent cleavage of C3. It is planned that this drug, named Compstatin (Potentia Pharmaceuticals), will soon enter phase 1 clinical trials for AMD [78].

a large number of technical difficulties, but some of the procedures that have been performed so far have been successful. The use of autologous RPE cells from aged donors has raised the question of whether a rejuvenating step should be introduced to enhance RPE cell function [6]. This can be performed by introducing a tissue culture step between the harvest and final transplantation procedure. A culture period will also allow the placement of the cells on a matrix, which can be used to replace a worn out Bruch's membrane. Further developments in this area are urgently needed, since this approach may also be beneficial for patients with dry AMD, for whom there are currently no available therapeutic options.

Summary for the Clinician

- Intravitreal injections of humanized antibodies to a variety of biologically active substances may selectively target mediators that play an important role in the pathogenesis of AMD.
- The use of antibodies against VEGF such as Lucentis and Avastin has revolutionized the treatment of wet AMD.
- The clinical use of a number of other antibodies (directed against TNF, the IL-2 receptor, C5) will be explored in the near future.
- Oligonucleotides directed against VEGF (Macugen) have already been approved for the treatment of wet AMD but are rapidly being superseded by the VEGF antibody preparations.

Summary for the Clinician

- Replacement of defective RPE cells and worn out Bruch's membrane is an option that is only performed in a few clinics around the world
- Translocation of a full-thickness (RPE, Bruch's membrane and choroid) graft can result in a functioning graft in patients with the dry form of AMD
- Transplantation of previously cultured autologous RPE cells is still being developed, and may also provide a treatment modality for patients with dry AMD

8.9   Retinal Transplantations

Cell replacement in AMD is primarily directed at replacing defective RPE cells. Rotation surgery for AMD involving relocation of the retina was reported as far back as the early 1990s [62]. Translocation of autologous Bruch's membrane, choriocapillaris, and choroid from the midperiphery to the macular area has shown the survival of such patches for up to four years after surgery in patients with neovascular AMD [61]. Recently, the same procedure was reported in patients with nonvascular AMD and was shown to be associated with a large number of complications and visual loss [49].

In view of these complications, a procedure where a sheet of RPE cells is transplanted has been favored. Transplantation of allogeneic or fetal RPE cells has often resulted in immunological rejection, and therefore most attention is focused on autologous transplantation [7]. Transplantation of autologous RPE cells in AMD faces

References

1. Ambati J, Anand A, Fernandez S et al. (2003) An animal model of age-related macular degeneration in senescent Ccl-2-or Ccr-2-deficient mice. Nat Med 9:1390–1397

2. Anderson DH, Mullins RF, Hageman GS et al. (2002) Perspective—A role for local inflammation in the formation of drusen in the aging eye. Am J Ophthalmol 134:411–431

3. Anderson DH, Talaga KC, Rivest AJ et al. (2004) Characterization of beta amyloid assemblies in drusen: the deposits associated with aging and age-related macular degeneration. Exp Eye Res 78:243–256

4. Apte RS, Richter J, Herndon J et al. (2006) Macrophages inhibit neovascularization in a murine model of age-related macular degeneration. Plos Medicine 3:1371–1381

5. Beatty S, Koh HH, Henson D et al. (2000) The role of oxidative stress in the pathogenesis of age-related macular degeneration. Surv Ophthalmol 45:115–134

6. Binder S, Stanzel BV, Krebs I et al. (2007) Transplantation of the RPE in AMD. Prog Retin Eye Res 26:516–554

7. Binder S, Stolba U, Krebs I et al. (2002) Transplantation of autologous retinal pigment epithelium in eyes with

foveal neovascularization resulting from age-related macular degeneration: a pilot study. Am J Ophthalmol 133:215–225

8. Boekhoorn SS, Vingerling JR, Witteman JCM et al. (2007) C-reactive protein level and risk of aging macula disorder— The Rotterdam study. Arch Ophthalmol 125:1396–1401

9. Bressler NM, Arnold J, Benchaboune M et al. (2002) Verteporfin therapy of subfoveal choroidal neovascularization in patients with age-related macular degeneration—Additional information regarding baseline lesion composition's impact on vision outcomes—TAP report No. 3. Arch Ophthalmol 120:1443–1454

10. Chaudhary V, Mao A, Hooper PL et al. (2007) Triamcinolone acetonide as adjunctive treatment to verteporfin in neovascular age-related macular degeneration—A prospective randomized trial. Ophthalmology 114:2183–2189

11. Chen L, Yang PZ, Kijlstra A (2002) Distribution, markers, and functions of retinal microglia. Ocul Immunol Inflamm 10:27–39

12. Chen L, Zwart R, Yang PZ et al. (2003) Macrophages and MHC class II positive dendritiform cells in the iris and choroid of the pig. Curr Eye Res 26:291–296

13. Cherepanoff S, Mitchell P, Wang JJ et al. (2006) Retinal autoantibody profile in early age-related macular degeneration: preliminary findings from the Blue Mountains Eye Study. Clin Experiment Ophthalmol 34:590 595

14. Chua B, Flood V, Rochtchina E et al. (2006) Dietary fatty acids and the 5-year incidence of age-related maculopathy. Arch Ophthalmol 124:981–986

15. Ciulla TA, Criswell MH, Danis RP et al. (2003) Choroidal neovascular membrane inhibition in a laser treated rat model with intraocular sustained release triamcinolone acetonide microimplants. Br J Ophthalmol 87:1032 1037

16. Dentchev T, Milam AH, Lee VMY et al. (2003) Amyloidbeta is found in drusen from some age-related macular degeneration retinas, but not in drusen from normal retinas. Mol Vis 9:184–190

17. Despriet DD, Bergen AA, Merriam JE et al. (2008) Comprehensive analysis of the candidate genes CCL2, CCR2, and TLR4 in age-related macular degeneration. Invest Ophthalmol Vis Sci 49:364–71

18. Donati G (2007) Emerging therapies for neovascular age-related macular degeneration: State of the art. Ophthalmologica 221:366–377

19. Ebrahem Q, Renganathan K, Sears J et al. (2006) Carboxyethylpyrrole oxidative protein modifications stimulate neovascularization: Implications for age-related macular degeneration. Proc Natl Acad Sci USA 103:13480–13484

20. Edwards AO, Ritter R, Abel KJ et al. (2005) Complement factor H polymorphism and age-related macular degeneration. Science 308:421–424

21. Epstein SE, Zhu JH, Burnett MS et al. (2000) Infection and atherosclerosis—Potential roles of pathogen burden and molecular mimicry. Arterioscler Thromb Vasc Biol 20:1417–1420

22. Espinosa-Heidmann DG, Suner IJ, Hernandez EP et al. (2003) Macrophage depletion diminishes lesion size and severity in experimental choroidal neovascularization. Invest Ophthalmol Vis Sci 44:3586–3592

23. Ferrara N, Gerber HP, LeCouter J (2003) The biology of VEGF and its receptors. Nat Med 9:669–676

24. Forrester JV, McMenamin PG, Holthouse I et al. (1994) Localization and characterization of major histocompatibility complex class II-positive cells in the posterior segment of the eye—implications for induction of autoimmune uveoretinitis. Invest Ophthalmol Vis Sci 35:64–77

25. Fukuoka Y, Strainic M, Medof ME (2003) Differential cytokine expression of human retinal pigment epithelial cells in response to stimulation by C5a. Clin Exp Immunol 131:248–253

26. Gehrs KM, Anderson DH, Johnson LV et al. (2006) Age-related macular degeneration—emerging pathogenetic and therapeutic concepts. Ann Med 38:450–471

27. Gold B, Merriam JE, Zernant J et al. (2006) Variation in factor B (BF) and complement component 2 (C2) genes is associated with age-related macular degeneration. Nat Genet 38:458–462

28. Gordon S, Taylor PR (2005) Monocyte and macrophage heterogeneity. Nat Rev Immunol 5:953–964

29. Gu XR, Meer SG, Miyagi M et al. (2003) Carboxyethylpyrrole protein adducts and autoantibodies, biomarkers for age-related macular degeneration. J Biol Chem 278:42027–42035

30. Gupta N, Brown KE, Milam AH (2003) Activated microglia in human retinitis pigmentosa, late-onset retinal degeneration, and age-related macular degeneration. Exp Eye Res 76:463–471

31. Hageman GS, Anderson DH, Johnson LV et al. (2005) A common haplotype in the complement regulatory gene factor H (HF1/CFH) predisposes individuals to age-related macular degeneration. Proc Natl Acad Sci USA 102:7227–7232

32. Hageman GS, Luthert PJ, Chong NHV et al. (2001) An integrated hypothesis that considers drusen as biomarkers of immune-mediated processes at the RPE-Bruch's membrane interface in aging and age-related macular degeneration. Prog Retin Eye Res 20:705–732

33. Haines JL, Hauser MA, Schmidt S et al. (2005) Complement factor H variant increases the risk of age-related macular degeneration. Science 308:419–421

34. Hammond BR, Wooten BR, Snodderly DM (1996) Cigarette smoking and retinal carotenoids: implications for age-related macular degeneration. Vision Res 36:3003–3009

35. Herbert AP, Deakin JA, Schmidt CQ et al. (2007) Structure shows that a glycosaminoglycan and protein recognition site in factor H is perturbed by age-related macular degeneration-linked single nucleotide polymorphism. J Biol Chem 282:18960–18968

36. Hollyfield JG, Bonilha VL, Rayborn ME et al. (2008) Oxidative damage-induced inflammation initiates age-related macular degeneration. Nat Med 14(2):194–198

37. Holtkamp GM, Kijlstra A, Peek R et al. (2001) Retinal pigment epithelium-immune system interactions: Cytokine production and cytokine-induced changes. Prog Retin Eye Res 20:29–48

38. Holtkamp GM, Van Rossem M, De Vos AF et al. (1998) Polarized secretion of IL-6 and IL-8 by human retinal pigment epithelial cells. Clin Exp Immunol 112:34–43

39. Hughes AE, Orr N, Patterson C et al. (2007) Neovascular age-related macular degeneration risk based on CFH, LOC387715/HTRA1, and smoking. Plos Med 4:1993–2000

40. Ishida O, Oku H, Ikeda T et al. (2003) Is *Chlamydia pneumoniae* infection a risk factor for age related macular degeneration? Br J Ophthalmol 87:523–524

41. Izumi-Nagai K, Nagai N, Ohgami K et al. (2007) Macular pigment lutein is antiinflammatory in preventing choroidal neovascularization. Arterioscler Thromb Vasc Biol 27:2555–2562

42. Jin XH, Ohgami K, Shiratori K et al. (2006) Inhibitory effects of lutein on endotoxin-induced uveitis in Lewis rats. Invest Ophthalmol Vis Sci 47:2562–2568

43. Joachim SC, Bruns K, Lackner KJ et al. (2007) Analysis of IgG antibody patterns against retinal antigens and antibodies to alpha-crystallin, GFAP, and alpha-enolase in sera of patients with "wet" age-related macular degeneration. Graefes Arch Clin Exp Ophthalmol 245:619–626

44. Johnson LV, Leitner WP, Rivest AJ et al. (2002) The Alzheimer's A beta-peptide is deposited at sites of complement activation in pathologic deposits associated with aging and age-related macular degeneration. Proc Natl Acad Sci USA 99:11830–11835

45. Johnson LV, Leitner WP, Staples MK et al. (2001) Complement activation and inflammatory processes in drusen formation and age related macular degeneration. Exp Eye Res 73:887–896

46. Johnson LV, Ozaki S, Staples MK et al. (2000) A potential role for immune complex pathogenesis in drusen formation. Exp Eye Res 70:441–449

47. Jonas JB, Kreissig I, Degenring R (2003) Intraocular pressure after intravitreal injection of triamcinolone acetonide. Br J Ophthalmol 87:24–27

48. Jonas JB, Kreissig I, Hugger P et al. (2003) Intravitreal triamcinolone acetonide for exudative age related macular degeneration. Br J Ophthalmol 87:462–468

49. Joussen AM, Joeres S, Fawzy N et al. (2007) Autologous translocation of the choroid and retinal pigment epithelium in patients with geographic atrophy. Ophthalmology 114:551–560

50. Kalayoglu MV, Bula D, Arroyo J et al. (2005) Identification of *Chlamydia pneumoniae* within human choroidal neovascular membranes secondary to age-related macular degeneration. Graefes Arch Clin Exp Ophthalmol 243:1080–1090

51. Kalayoglu MV, Galvan C, Mahdi OS et al. (2003) Serological association between *Chlamydia pneumoniae* infection and age-related macular degeneration. Arch Ophthalmol 121:478–482

52. Kassoff A, Kassoff J, Buehler J et al. (2001) A randomized, placebo-controlled, clinical trial of high-dose supplementation with vitamins C and E, beta carotene, and zinc for age-related macular degeneration and vision loss—AREDS Report No. 8. Arch Ophthalmol 119:1417–1436

53. Kelly J, Khan AA, Yin J et al. (2007) Senescence regulates macrophage activation and angiogenic fate at sites of tissue injury in mice. J Clin Invest 117:3421–3426

54. Kessler W, Jantos CA, Dreier J et al. (2006) *Chlamydia pneumoniae* is not detectable in subretinal neovascular membranes in the exudative stage of age-related macular degeneration. Acta Ophthalmol Scand 84:333–337

55. Klein R, Peto T, Bird A et al. (2004) The epidemiology of age-related macular degeneration. Am J Ophthalmol 137:486–495

56. Klein RJ, Zeiss C, Chew EY et al. (2005) Complement factor H polymorphism in age-related macular degeneration. Science 308:385–389

57. Kliffen M, Sharma HS, Mooy CM et al. (1997) Increased expression of angiogenic growth factors in age-related maculopathy. Br J Ophthalmol 81:154–162

58. Kvanta A, Algvere PV, Berglin L et al. (1996) Subfoveal fibrovascular membranes in age-related macular degeneration express vascular endothelial growth factor. Invest Ophthalmol Vis Sci 37:1929–1934

59. Lee J, Freeman WR, Azen SP et al. (2007) Prospective, randomized clinical trial of intravitreal triamcinolone treatment of neovascular age-related macular degeneration—One-year results. Retina J Ret Vit Dis 27:1205–1213

60. Luibl V, Isas JM, Kayed R et al. (2006) Drusen deposits associated with aging and age-related macular degeneration contain nonfibrillar amyloid oligomers. J Clin Invest 116:378–385

61. Maaijwee K, Heimann H, Missotten T et al. (2007) Retinal pigment epithelium and choroid translocation in patients with exudative age-related macular degeneration: long-term results. Graefes Arch Clin Exp Ophthalmol 245:1681–1689

62. Machemer R, Steinhorst UH (1993) Retinal separation, retinotomy, and macular relocation. 2. A surgical approach

for age-related macular degeneration. Graefes Arch Clin Exp Ophthalmol 231:635–641

63. McLaughlin BJ, Fan W, Zheng JJ et al. (2003) Novel role for a complement regulatory protein (CD46) in retinal pigment epithelial adhesion. Invest Ophthalmol Vis Sci 44:3669–3674

64. Miller DM, Espinos-Heidmann DG, Legra J et al. (2004) The association of prior cytomegalovirus infection with neovascular age-related macular degeneration. Am J Ophthalmol 138:323–328

65. Moeller SM, Parekh N, Tinker L et al. (2006) Associations between intermediate age-related macular degeneration and lutein and zeaxanthin in the carotenoids in age-related eye disease study (CAREDS)—Ancillary study of the women's health initiative. Arch Ophthalmol 124:1151–1162

66. Monk PN, Scola AM, Madala P et al. (2007) Function, structure and therapeutic potential of complement C5a receptors. Br J Pharmacol 152:429–448

67. Mori K, Gehlbach P, Yamamoto S et al. (2002) AAV-Mediated gene transfer of pigment epithelium-derived factor inhibits choroidal neovascularization. Invest Ophthalmol Vis Sci 43:1994–2000

68. Nauta AJ, Daha MR, van Kooten C et al. (2003) Recognition and clearance of apoptotic cells: a role for complement and pentraxins. Trends Immunol 24:148–154

69. Newsome DA, Hewitt AT, Huh W et al. (1987) Detection of specific extracellular-matrix molecules in drusen, Bruch's membrane, and ciliary body. Am J Ophthalmol 104:373–381

70. Ng EWM, Shima DT, Calias P et al. (2006) Pegaptanib, a targeted anti-VEGF aptamer for ocular vascular disease. Nat Rev Drug Discov 5:123–132

71. Nozaki M, Raisler BJ, Sakurai E et al. (2006) Drusen complement components C3a and C5a promote choroidal neovascularization. Proc Natl Acad Sci USA 103:2328–2333

72. Nussenblatt RB, Ferris F (2007) Age-related macular degeneration and the immune response: implications for therapy. Am J Ophthalmol 144:618–626

73. Patel N, Ohbayashi M, Nugent AK et al. (2005) Circulating anti-retinal antibodies as immune markers in age-related macular degeneration. Immunology 115:422–430

74. Penfold PL, Madigan MC, Gillies MC et al. (2001) Immunological and aetiological aspects of macular degeneration. Prog Retin Eye Res 20:385–414

75. Penn JS, Rajaratnam VS, Collier RJ et al. (2001) The effect of an angiostatic steroid on neovascularization in a rat model of retinopathy of prematurity. Invest Ophthalmol Vis Sci 42:283–290

76. Radisavljevic Z, Avraham H, Avraham S (2000) Vascular endothelial growth factor up-regulates ICAM-1 expression via the phosphatidylinositol 3 OH-kinase/AKT/nitric oxide pathway and modulates migration of brain microvascular endothelial cells. J Biol Chem 275:20770–20774

77. Richer S, Stiles W, Statkute L et al. (2004) Double-masked, placebo-controlled, randomized trial of lutein and antioxidant supplementation in the intervention of atrophic age-related macular degeneration: the Veterans LAST study (Lutein Antioxidant Supplementation Trial). Optometry 75:216–230

78. Ricklin D, Lambris JD (2007) Complement-targeted therapeutics. Nat Biotechnol 25:1265–1275

79. Robman L, Mahdi OS, Wang JJ et al. (2007) Exposure to *Chlamydia pneumoniae* infection and age-related macular degeneration: the Blue Mountains Eye Study. Invest Ophthalmol Vis Sci 48:4007–4011

80. Rosenfeld PJ, Brown DM, Heier JS et al. (2006) Ranibizumab for neovascular age-related macular degeneration. N Engl J Med 355:1419–1431

81. SanGiovanni JP, Chew EY (2005) The role of omega-3 long-chain polyunsaturated fatty acids in health and disease of the retina. Prog Retin Eye Res 24:87–138

82. Seregard S, Algvere PV, Berglin L (1994) Immunohistochemical characterization of surgically removed subfoveal fibrovascular membranes. Graefes Arch Clin Exp Ophthalmol 232:325–329

83. Shankar A, Mitchell P, Rochtchina E et al. (2007) Association between circulating white blood cell count and long-term incidence of age-related macular degeneration—The Blue Mountains Eye Study. Am J Epidemiol 165:375–382

84. Spaide RF, Laud K, Fine HF et al. (2006) Intravitreal bevacizumab treatment of choroidal neovascularization secondary to age-related macular degeneration. Retina J Ret Vit Dis 26:383–390

85. Sutter FKP, Gillies MC (2003) Pseudo-endophthalmitis after intravitreal injection of triamcinolone. Br J Ophthalmol 87:972–974

86. Tezel TH, Bodek E, Sonmez K et al. (2007) Targeting tissue factor for immunotherapy of choroidal neovascularization by intravitreal delivery of factor VII-Fc chimeric antibody. Ocul Immunol Inflamm 15:3–10

87. Vanderschaft TL, Mooy CM, Debruijn WC et al. (1993) Early stages of age-related macular degeneration—an immunofluorescence and electron-microscopy study. Br J Ophthalmol 77:657–661

88. Vogt SD, Barnum SR, Curcio CA et al. (2006) Distribution of complement anaphylatoxin receptors and membrane-bound regulators in normal human retina. Exp Eye Res 83:834–840

89. Wang JJ, Mitchell P, Smith W et al. (2003) Systemic use of anti-inflammatory medications and age-related maculopathy: the Blue Mountains Eye Study. Ophthalmic Epidemiol 10:37–48

90. Wang YS, Friedrichs U, Eichler W et al. (2002) Inhibitory effects of triamcinolone acetonide on bFGF-induced migration and tube formation in choroidal microvascular endothelial cells. Graefes Arch Clin Exp Ophthalmol 240:42–48

91. Zhou JL, Jang YP, Kim SR et al. (2006) Complement activation by photooxidation products of A2E, a lipofuscin constituent of the retinal pigment epithelium. Proc Natl Acad Sci USA 103:16182–16187

Chapter 9

Patterns of Retinal Vascular Involvement in the Diagnosis of Retinal Vasculitis

9

Miles R. Stanford, Rashmi Mathew

Core Messages

- Identification of which retinal vessels are predominantly involved is key in establishing the underlying aetiology of RV.
- Retinal arteriole involvement is almost always due to intraocular infection (commonly viral retinitis, toxoplasma); syphilis may involve retinal arterioles, but can also affect other vessels.
- Retinal vein involvement is seen in Behçet's disease, sarcoidosis, multiple sclerosis, inflammatory bowel disease, seronegative arthropathy and in isolated idiopathic RV.
- Significant retinal ischaemia is seen in tuberculosis, Eales disease, Behçet's disease and ischaemic idiopathic isolated retinal vasculitis.

- Neovascularisation may occur in the presence or absence of retinal capillary closure; in the latter case, adequate immunosuppression will suppress the neovascular process.
- Branch retinal vein occlusion in the presence of intraocular inflammation is due to Behçet's disease, until proven otherwise. It has been reported in patients with sarcoidosis and tuberculosis.
- Few pathological studies are available on eyes with RV. Those that are available tend to have been removed for end-stage disease, and the pathological picture may be altered by the immunosuppression that the patient has received. Accordingly, little is known about the early processes underlying RV.

9.1 Introduction

Retinal vasculitis is a generic name for the clinical syndrome of intraocular inflammation coupled with involvement of retinal vessels. As such, it encompasses a broad spectrum of different diseases ranging from intraocular infection to malignancy. Most commonly, however, it is idiopathic, although systemic inflammatory diseases such as multiple sclerosis and sarcoidosis may develop with time.

Confusion in the nomenclature often arises, as the term vasculitis usually refers pathologically to a type III hypersensitivity reaction with deposition of immune complexes within the vessel wall and resultant fibrinoid necrosis. Although this pathological process may occur in retinal vessels in conditions such as Wegener's granulomatosis, polyarteritis nodosa and systemic lupus erythematosus, it is rare to find accompanying intraocular inflammation. Accordingly, the diagnosis of retinal vasculitis (RV) is a clinical one, which can be complimented by fundus fluorescein angiography (FFA) where either vascular leakage and staining of retinal vessel walls representing localised inflammatory breakdown of the inner blood retinal barrier or vascular closure resulting from inflammation may be observed. Either pattern can be associated with retinal neovascularisation. RV usually affects the retinal venous system, but arterioles and capillaries can also be involved. Given the wide variety of diseases that give rise to the clinical picture of RV, a careful history and examination are required to achieve a diagnosis. Investigations should be tailored to the individual patient's symptoms and signs, as numerous studies have shown that little information is gained by blind investigation of the patient [1]. A high index of suspicion for infection and malignancy is required, as these conditions can be made worse by inappropriate treatment.

In this chapter, we will concentrate on the clinicopathological aspects of RV that occur in different diseases, and why these differences help in their differential diagnosis. We do not intend to evaluate the management of these disorders, as this is a rapidly changing field and there is little evidence from randomised trials to provide guidance.

9.2 Pathology of Retinal Vasculitis

9.2.1 General Pathology of Retinal Vessels

Little is known about the pathology of retinal vasculitis, as it is a disease that primarily affects the young, and enucleated eyes or those taken at post mortem tend to have end-stage, chronic disease. This means that early changes relating to pathogenesis cannot be observed and that treatment will have modified the pattern of inflammation. Key events in the course of retinal vasculitis always involve the breakdown of the inner blood–retinal barrier, but despite decades of clinical and experimental research, very little is known about this fundamental step. Simultaneously, there is a diapedesis of inflammatory cells into the retina, which may remain in a perivascular location (giving rise to signs of periphlebitis), or may invade the retina (retinal infiltrates). The pathological outcome of this initial insult around retinal vascular endothelial cells is that the vessels either continue to leak, with the production of retinal oedema, or they occlude, often with the neovascular and fibrotic consequences of this change. Fortunately, current treatment may reverse the barrier breakdown with resolution of symptoms and clinical signs. The pathological changes that occur in the healing phase of this inflammatory response often cause gliosis of retinal vascular walls, giving rise to the clinical appearance of peripheral venous sheathing. This term encompasses four entities: congenital sheathing (persistent embryonic connective tissue), post-inflammatory sheathing (perivascular gliosis), "halo" sheathing of venous sclerosis, and periphlebitic sheathing (active periphlebitis). Sheathing is actually collagenous thickening of the vessel wall due to prior chronic flow impairment, either from associated arteriolar sclerosis (as in branch retinal vein occlusions) or from perivascular inflammation.

9.2.2 Pathology of Retinal Vessels in Specific Diseases

9.2.2.1 Behçet's Disease

Charteris et al. reported on the histopathology of five cases of Behçet's disease (BD) who had severe panuveitis at the time of enucleation [2]. They demonstrated intramural and perivascular infiltrates of CD4+ T lymphocytes. No CD8 T lymphocytes were identified and B-lymphocytes were an infrequent finding. No complement or immunoglobulin deposition was identified. They concluded that the high proportion of CD4+ T lymphocytes and the lack of immunoglobulin or complement deposition

implicated a central role for cell-mediated immunity in the pathophysiology of BD. The findings of this study were reinforced by a further report of the pathology of the eyes from a patient who died from the systemic complications of BD, which showed marked hyaline thickening of the retinal and optic nerve vessels. The vessels had an intramural and perivascular infiltrate of T lymphocytes which stained positively for CD4 and IL-2 receptor surface markers [3].

George et al. also found T lymphocytes to be the predominant inflammatory cell type in ocular BD [4]. However, in contrast to prior reports, they found focal aggregates of B-lymphocytes and many plasma cells in the retina. In addition, the vascular endothelium showed extensive expression of adhesion molecules and major histocompatibility class (MHC) II antigens. Occluded vessels were shown to contain perivascular infiltrates of mononuclear cells, and proliferation of vascular endothelial cells leading to varying degrees of obliteration.

Much discussion has centred around whether the pathophysiological process in BD involves immune-complex deposition or cell-mediated immunity. The predominant ocular infiltrating cells in the above studies of patients with BD were immunocompetent T-helper cells and plasma cells. The abundant expression of MHC class II antigens suggests that there is active presentation of antigen to CD4 T cells, which plays a major role in cell-mediated immunity. However, as the eyes obtained in these studies were late stage, it may be that the pathological picture represented a steady state immune reaction rather than being indicative of early disease. The abundance of these CD4 T cells and the relative lack of T-suppressor cells (CD8) may lead to B-cell stimulation and polyclonal B-cell activation, explaining the numerous plasma cells which were observed in the above study. This local production of antibodies may lead to immune-complex deposition. It is likely therefore that the immunological mechanisms underlying the pathophysiology of BD involve all parts of the immune response, with certain elements being more prominent at different times.

9.2.2.2 Tuberculosis

In 1911, Axenfeld and Stock were the first to propose a tuberculous cause for retinal periphlebitis [5], and Fleischer was the first to report pathologic changes in the retina consistent with tuberculous infection [6]. The retina is rarely affected by *M. tuberculosis* and is most commonly affected secondarily from adjacent choroidal lesions. Donahue reported finding seven cases of periphlebitis among 10,524 patients with systemic TB.

In 1935, Gilbert reported finding tubercle bacilli surrounding a retinal vein in a patient with retinal periphlebitis [8]. However, neither caseous necrosis nor acid-fast bacilli were found. The DNA of *M. tuberculosis* has also been detected in aqueous or vitreous humour taps and in epiretinal membranes.

Although a diagnosis of TB is not always confirmed, many clinicians attribute retinal periphlebitis to direct infection because of the response to antituberculous therapy [9, 10]. In addition, patients with retinal periphlebitis may show evidence of active or healed pulmonary tuberculosis (TB). Occasionally treatment with oral corticosteroids for retinal vasculitis may result in a disseminated TB, reaffirming the belief that TB may be the underlying cause.

It is highly debatable as to whether the vasculitis results from the presence of tubercle bacilli or whether it represents a hypersensitivity reaction to tubercular antigens. This latter mechanism is thought to underlie the pathophysiology of Eales disease. Retinal periphlebitis is a prominent finding in early Eales' disease, but most patients present with the late complications of the disease. Few histopathological studies of eyes with Eales disease exist [11,12,13]. In those that are available, the uniform finding has been lymphocytic infiltration in and around retinal veins. Endothelial proliferation in the vessel wall with narrowing or obliteration of the lumen has also been noted. Although the absence of giant cells and caseation does not exclude the diagnosis of TB, there is little evidence to support a direct infection by tubercle bacilli in the retinas of patients with Eales disease.

9.2.2.3 Sarcoidosis

The pathological findings in the eyes of patients with ocular sarcoidosis reflect those of systemic disease. Prominent features include perivenular and venular invasion by inflammatory cells and obliteration of the lumen by the inflammatory reaction. The retinal venules show moderate to marked lymphocytic and histiocytic infiltration. Vessels can also be completely occluded by noncaseating granulomata [14].

Chan et al. showed that 90% of the T lymphocytes were of the T-helper variety, again pointing to cell-mediated immunity in the pathophysiology of sarcoidosis [15].

9.2.2.4 Multiple Sclerosis

In a post-mortem examination, Arnold et al. examined 47 patients with multiple sclerosis (MS) and found seven eyes with periphlebitis [16]. On gross examination, periphlebitis appeared as a segmental fluffy white haziness parallelling and in some regions obscuring vessels in the peripheral retina. Arterioles were not visibly affected. Microscopically, a segmental perivenous lymphoplasmocytic infiltrate involving the anterior and posterior retinal veins was seen. In two cases, the infiltrate had subtle granulomatous features. The perivenular sheathing is similar to the perivenular cellular infiltrate in the CNS of MS patients [17].

9.2.2.5 Idiopathic Isolated Retinal Vasculitis

Idiopathic isolated retinal vasculitis is an inflammatory condition affecting retinal veins. It encompasses clinical entities such as intermediate uveitis and pars planitis, as well as posterior uveitis without choroiditis. The majority of the pathological findings in this condition are derived from observations of eyes taken from patients with pars planitis. These showed inflammation that was confined to the vitreous and retina, with no uveal inflammation. Retinal veins contained intramural inflammatory cells which were predominantly T-helper cells, whilst arteries were spared [18, 19]. Venular sheathing has been found in up to 50% of patients [20]. Often there was pathological evidence of neovascularisation within snowbanks.

9.2.2.6 Acute Retinal Necrosis

Acute retinal necrosis is a fulminant obliterative vasculitis usually associated with infection of the retina by DNA viruses (herpes simplex, varicella, cytomegalovirus and Epstein–Barr virus). One of the cardinal clinical signs is occlusion of retinal arteries [21]. Culbertson et al. described the histopathological findings of an enucleated eye secondary to acute retinal necrosis, which had no perception of light acuity after only nine days of disease [22]. They found sharp demarcation between involved and uninvolved retina, which is consistent with viral cell-to-cell transmission. The arteries were heavily infiltrated and surrounded by inflammatory cells. Cellular thrombi filled the branch arteries near the surface of the disc. Large numbers of lymphocytes, macrophages and polymorphonuclear leucocytes were seen, which suggested an active inflammatory and cell-mediated response to the offending agent. Eosinophilic intranuclear inclusions were detected on electron microscopy. These findings have also been confirmed in other pathological studies.

9.2.2.7 Sympathetic Ophthalmia

Histologically, sympathetic ophthalmia is characterised by diffuse chronic granulomatous panuveitis, with a cellular infiltrate composed predominantly of lymphocytes and scattered nests of epithelioid cells. In the infiltrate there may be numerous eosinophils, but plasma cells and polymorphonuclear leucocytes are rarely present. A study of a hundred cases of sympathetic ophthalmia looking specifically at atypical features showed retinal perivasculitis [23], mostly around venules in 55% of cases, and marked perivasculitis in 31%. There was no preferential location. There was mild retinal inflammation unrelated to perivasculitis in 18% of cases. The cells were mostly lymphocytes and occasionally polymorphonuclear leucocytes. Retinal involvement was not related to the degree of choroidal inflammation.

It can be seen from the above pathological studies that the histological features of the diseases associated with retinal vasculitis closely mimic their clinical features. In particular, there is value in determining whether the inflammatory focus is predominantly centred on retinal arteries (acute retinal necrosis) or retinal veins (Behçet's, sarcoidosis, MS, etc.).

Summary for the Clinician

- Few pathological studies exist of eyes with RV
- Studies are usually carried out on eyes with end-stage disease, where the patient has been on long-term immunosuppression, which will have modified the pathological response
- Little is known about the early immunopathological events in RV
- In the majority of eyes studied, the disease seems to be mediated through T-cell dominant processes

---

9.3 Clinical Features of Retinal Vasculitis

The most important clinical clues can be derived from identifying the retinal vessels that are involved in the inflammatory process (see Table 9.1). Thus, inflammation of the retinal arteries (periarteritis) is almost always due to a viral retinitis, toxoplasmosis or systemic vasculitis. Syphilis can cause inflammation of any sort or calibre of retinal vessel. Predominant involvement of retinal veins occurs in Behçet's disease, sarcoidosis, multiple sclerosis, inflammatory bowel disease, seronegative arthropathies, and in idiopathic isolated disease. Periphlebitis defined as a focal fluffy white cuffing of the retinal veins, which is characterised by focal leakage of fluorescein at these sites of inflammation, usually occurs in sarcoidosis and in TB. Intraretinal infiltrates are characteristic of acute bacterial endophthalmitis, but in the absence of infection are

pathognomonic for Behçet's disease. Cotton wool spots are also found in association with systemic vasculitides. Swelling of the optic nerve head is a common nonspecific finding related to the intraocular inflammation but may also represent infiltrative disease of the nerve itself.

9.3.1 Primary, Idiopathic, Isolated RV

Isolated idiopathic RV is a sight-threatening inflammatory eye disease mainly affecting the young. In a study by Graham et al., two-thirds of patients with idiopathic RV were under the age of 40. However, it can also be asymptomatic if the peripheral retinal vasculature is only involved, such cases usually being identified through routine visits to the optometrist. Patients mostly complain of painless blurring of vision with floaters. Symptoms of anterior uveitis are uncommon unless there is spill-over of the inflammation into the anterior segment.

RV is one of the cardinal signs of posterior segment inflammation. It classically affects the venules. A review of the retinal signs in 67 patients with idiopathic RV showed that "sheathing" or "cuffing" of the retinal vasculature was the most prevalent finding, affecting 64% of patients, followed by macular oedema in 60% [24].

RV is characterised by increased permeability of the retinal vasculature with extravasation of inflammatory cells, leading to cystoid macular oedema (CMO) and vitritis. Alternatively, it may be occlusive in nature, causing retinal ischaemia with new vessel formation and vitreous haemorrhage [25]. Thus RV can be broadly classified into nonischaemic and ischaemic forms. Signs of occlusive RV include retinal haemorrhages, cotton wool spots, retinal and optic nerve head oedema. Venous occlusion results in capillary nonperfusion, ischaemia and, depending on the extent of nonperfusion, neovascularisation. Vascular leakage on the other hand leads to retinal swelling and exudation.

It is important to detect signs of retinal ischaemia, as the prognosis varies between the two forms of the disease. In ischaemic RV, areas of retinal capillary nonperfusion are seen either as large areas of capillary drop-out (Fig. 9.1) or as an irregular enlargement of the foveal avascular zone. In a review of 345 angiograms of 135 patients with chronic posterior uveitis, 12 patients (four sarcoid, four Behçet's, four idiopathic) were identified as having macular ischaemia on FFA, all of whom had a poor visual outcome [26]. Whilst reports from tertiary clinics are subject to referral bias, Palmer et al. showed that 33% of their population had ischaemic changes [27]. In a similar group of patients, George et al. found ischaemic changes in two-thirds of patients [1].

Table 9.1 Ophthalmological features of conditions associated with retinal vasculitis

	Idiopathic isolated RV	Behçet's disease	Sarcoid	MS	Sympathetic ophthalmia	Eales' disease	Tuberculosis	Toxoplasmosis	Syphilis	Viral
Periarteritis	−	−	−	++	−	−	−	+	++	++
Periphlebitis	+	++	+++	++	+	+	++	+	+	−
Macular oedema	++	+	++	−	+	−	+	-	+	
Peripheral venous sheathing	++			++	−	−	+	++	+	−
Retinal vein occlusion	−	+	+/−	+/−	−	+ (Peripheral)	+	Rare	Rare	−
Neovascularisation	++	++	+	+	−	++	+	Rare	Rare	−
Disc swelling	++	+	+	+	+	−	+	−	+	+
Pigment epithelial disease	−	−	+	−	++	−	+	++	++	−
FFA features										
- Diffuse micro-vascular leakage	++	++	−	++	+	−	++	−	++	−
- Focal leakage	−	−	++	+	−	−	−	+	−	+
- Capillary closure	−	++	+	++	−	+++	+	-	+	++
- Neovascularisation	+	++	++	+	−	++	+	Rare	Rare	−
Other		Retinal infiltrates	Candle-wax drippings		Dalen–Fuchs nodules; Retinal detachment			Kyrieleis plaques		Retinitis; Retinal detachment

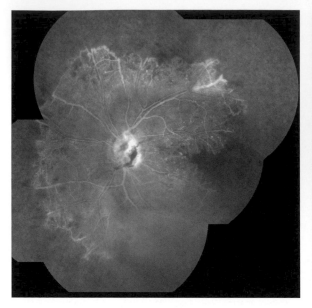

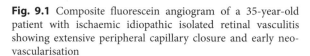

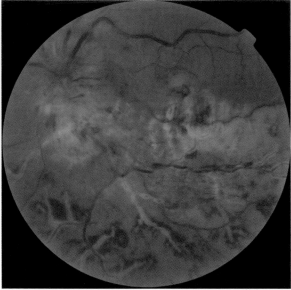

Fig. 9.1 Composite fluorescein angiogram of a 35-year-old patient with ischaemic idiopathic isolated retinal vasculitis showing extensive peripheral capillary closure and early neovascularisation

Fig. 9.2 Colour fundus photograph of a 42-year-old patient with Behçet's disease showing an inferotemporal branch vein occlusion. This was ischaemic on fluorescein angiography, and the patient subsequently developed new vessels elsewhere

9.3.2   Systemic Disease and RV

9.3.2.1   Behçet's Disease

Behçet's disease (BD) is a multisystem chronic inflammatory disorder. In BD, the predominant clinical symptoms are related to inflammation of the veins, and this is applicable to the eye too. In 1985 the International Study Group for BD outlined diagnostic criteria for BD [28]. Ocular inflammation is one of the major criteria for the diagnosis of BD and occurs in up to 85% of patients, and retinal lesions are present in 50–93% of those with ocular involvement.

In the absence of intraretinal infection, the presence of yellow-white retinal infiltrates is pathognomonic for BD. Recurrent, ischaemic, inflammatory branch retinal vein occlusions (Fig. 9.2) in the presence of intraocular inflammation are due to BD until proven otherwise. Neovascularisation of the disc and elsewhere secondary to retinal ischaemia with ensuing vitreous haemorrhage is also a common finding.

FFA findings are characterised by diffuse microvascular leakage and vascular staining. Capillary closure occurs secondary to vein occlusions, resulting in retinal ischaemia and subsequent retinal and disc neovascularisation.

In an analysis of the retinal findings in 39 patients with Behçet's disease, the most prevalent ophthalmological findings were diffuse capillary leakage (100%), branch retinal vein occlusions (64%) and retinal infiltrates (33%). Retinal neovascularisation occurred in less than 10%. Extensive capillary closure was demonstrated in those with recurrent retinal vein occlusions [24].

9.3.2.2   Eales Disease

Eales disease classically presents with repeated vitreous haemorrhage in young adult men. Men account for 80–90% of cases. Fundal examination in the early phase of the disease reveals retinal periphlebitis, predominantly in the peripheral fundus and inflammatory vein occlusions, which are usually multiple. At the time of presentation the contralateral eye is involved in 50% of cases. Ultimately the involvement becomes bilateral in 80% of cases.

Eales disease starts with active periphlebitis. The inflamed venous walls stain on fluorescein angiography and have narrowed lumens. The segmental venous inflammation produces varying degrees of venous occlusion, from slight narrowing to complete closure and engorgement of the capillary beds. Repeated venular occlusions can cause widespread retinal ischaemia, which can lead to new vessel formation. New blood vessels typically appear in a sea-fan formation with looping. These are the most common sources of repeated vitreous haemorrhage in Eales. It should be noted that not all cases develop neovascular lesions. Recanalisation of inflamed venules, veno-venous capillary shunts and gradual degeneration of the retina often lead to stabilisation of a decompensated circulation.

9.3.2.3 Tuberculosis

Tuberculosis (TB) of the retina is a rare phenomenon and is always due to haematogenous spread. The most common retinal presentation is periphlebitis, but it may also result in vein occlusions, peripheral retinal closure and new vessel formation. Tuberculous RV is not characteristic, and unless choroidal tubercles are present, the fundal appearance (Fig. 9.3) may be similar to that seen in sarcoidosis, Behçets disease or isolated retinal vasculitis, and so may be misdiagnosed [29]. A definitive diagnosis of ocular TB requires the identification of *Mycobacterium tuberculosis*, which is often difficult to obtain. Hence it is often a presumed diagnosis, even in the presence of systemic TB.

9.3.2.4 Sarcoidosis

Sarcoidosis is an idiopathic granulomatous multisystem disorder. Ocular involvement occurs in 26–38% of patients and may be the initial manifestation in 10–20% of cases [30, 31]. Sarcoidosis is among the commonest causes of RV. Periphlebitis is the most common fundal feature (Fig. 9.4a and b) and is reported in up to 50% of patients [32]. Active periphlebitis appears clinically as a fluffy white haziness surrounding the blood column.

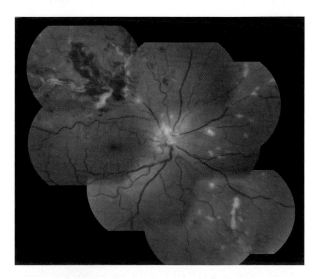

Fig. 9.3 Composite colour photograph of a 24-year-old patient with ocular tuberculosis. Note the haemorrhage in the superotemporal quadrant and the widespread perivenular infiltration

Involvement is patchy, with irregular extension outside the vessel wall. It represents a chronic inflammatory cell infiltrate within and surrounding the vein wall, which may resolve without sequelae or may be replaced by venous sclerosis. In sarcoidosis, the RV tends to be focal or segmental and involves small branch veins in the equatorial fundus, with or without vascular narrowing. Other retinal manifestations include segmental venular cuffing, sheathing and perivenous exudation, referred to as candle-wax drippings (tache de bougie), which represent non-necrotising granulomatous inflammation. This feature is not pathognomic for sarcoidosis, and can be found in syphilis, tuberculosis and Behçet's disease. Periphlebitis in the presence of choroidal or retinal pigment epithelial disease also points strongly towards sarcoidosis-related RV. Macular oedema is the most frequent and sight-threatening consequence of sarcoid uveitis. Retinal vein occlusion is rare in sarcoid and partly serves to distinguish it from BD. Approximately 15% of patients with posterior uveitis due to sarcoidosis will develop neovascularisation, which may occur in the presence or absence of retinal ischaemia.

Fundus fluorescein angiogram shows venule wall staining, focal leakage, capillary closure, cystoid macular oedema and neovascularisation. In a subgroup analysis of idiopathic RV, the most prevalent findings in sarcoidosis were retinal periphlebitis associated with focal leakage of fluorescein, which occurred in 11 patients (65%). Only three patients in this group developed retinal new vessels [24]. It has been reported that retinal involvement has a 35% risk of being associated with central nervous system or neurological problems [30].

9.3.2.5 Multiple Sclerosis

Multiple sclerosis (MS) is an idiopathic demyelinating disorder with ocular manifestations. The retinal vasculitis that is observed in MS is usually mild, commonly asymptomatic, and manifests as peripheral venous sheathing (Fig. 9.5). However, there is confusion in the nomenclature applied to this in the literature, with some authors using retinal periphlebitis interchangeably with retinal venous sheathing. This type of RV is quite characteristic of MS and is found in 8–18% of patients [16, 33]. The RV is transient and can completely resolve. It has been suggested that virtually all MS patients will have had RV at some point during their disease [34] The prevalence of RV is higher in hospital patients than those in rehabilitation centres, where MS is likely to be in a stable state; suggesting that retinal vascular involvement correlated with disease activity [35]. On FFA, patchy perivascular cuffing with leakage indicates activity, whereas venule

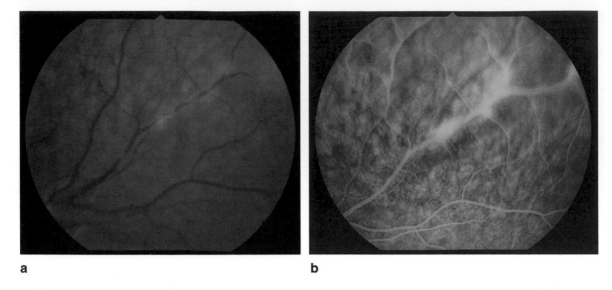

a   b

Fig. 9.4 a Colour photograph of a peripheral retinal vein in a 29-year-old patient with sarcoidosis; note the presence of periphlebitis.
b Fluorescein angiogram of the same vessel showing focal leakage in the same area

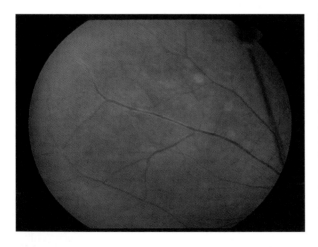

9.3.3   Retinal Vasculitis Associated with Infection

9.3.3.1   Viral Retinitis

Retinal involvement in systemic viral infection typically manifests as a necrotising retinitis with secondary retinal vasculitis. The prominent findings in acute retinal necrosis (ARN) include a severe, occlusive vasculitis that primarily involves the arteries of the retina (Fig. 9.6), and a discrete full-thickness necrotising retinitis. In the majority of cases, rhegmatogenous retinal detachment occurs as a late complication. The key to a good visual outcome is prompt accurate diagnosis. Bilateral involvement occurs in approximately one-third of patients, but both eyes may not be affected simultaneously. There is a bimodal distribution in the ages of the affected patients, with the peaks at about 20 and 50 years of age. The retinal vasculitis is manifested ophthalmoscopically by narrowing and sheathing of the larger vessels, especially in the mid-periphery, with accompanying areas of necrosis. One feature of ARN syndrome that sets it apart from most other types of infectious and inflammatory retinal conditions is the frequent development of full-thickness retinal holes. In HIV patients, a microvasculopathy consisting of cotton wool spots and intraretinal haemorrhages also occurs and is thought to be due to either localised damage to the retinal vascular endothelium by immune complex formation, direct infection of the retinal vascular

Fig. 9.5 Colour fundus photograph in the superotemporal quadrant of a 33-year-old lady with relapsing–remitting multiple sclerosis. Note the extensive perivenular sheathing

wall whitening with no leakage represents chronic sclerotic change [36].

Although rare, MS patients can also develop peripheral retinal neovascularisation. The recognition of ocular disease is important, as it may precede development of neurological signs and appears to signify a worse prognosis for the patient's systemic disease. In longitudinal studies of patients with pars planitis, 8–15% of patients went on to develop MS and 16–22% developed either MS or optic neuritis within 7.5 years [37,38,39].

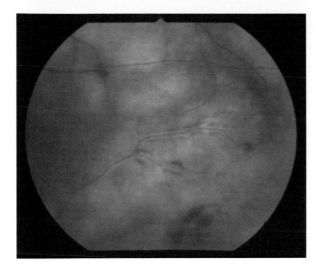

Fig. 9.6 Colour fundus photograph of the temporal periphery of the left eye, showing extensive areas of retinal necrosis. This patient was positive for herpes zoster by PCR of a vitreous specimen; note the preferential involvement of the retinal arterioles

endothelium by the virus with subsequent arteriolar occlusion, or abnormalities of blood viscosity [40].

9.3.3.2 Syphilis

The incidence of syphilis has markedly increased since the mid-1980s. As the ophthalmological manifestations of syphilis are protean, syphilis needs to be excluded in any patient with uveitis or retinal vasculitis. Retinal vascular changes are common in ocular syphilis; the commonest change being arterial involvement, but concomitant involvement of both arteries and veins and isolated periphlebitis has also been reported [41,42, 43,44].

Summary for the Clinician

- Predominant retinal arteriole involvement is seen in viral retinitis, toxoplasmosis and occasionally syphilis
- All other causes of RV affect retinal veins
- Fluorescein angiography may show leakage, closure and neovascularisation
- In the absence of endophthalmitis, retinal infiltrates are pathognomonic of Behçet's disease
- Branch retinal vein occlusion in an eye with posterior uveitis is due to Behçet's disease until proven otherwise

References

1. George RK, Walton RC, Whitcup SM et al. (1996) Primary retinal vasculitis: Systemic association and diagnostic value. Ophthalmology 103(3):384–389
2. Charteris DG, Champ C, Rosenthal AR et al. (1992) Behçet's disease: activated T lymphocytes in retinal perivasculitis. Br J Ophthalmol 76(8):499–501
3. Charteris DG, Barton K, McCartney AC et al. (1992) CD4+ lymphocyte involvement in ocular Behçet's disease. Autoimmunity 12(3):201–206
4. George RK, Chan CC, Whitcup SM et al. (1997) Ocular immunopathology of Behçet's disease. Surv Ophthalmol 42(2):157–162
5. Axenfeld T, Stock W (1911) Ueber die Bedeutung der Tuberkulose in der Aetiologie der intraokularen Hamorrhagien und der Proliferierenden veranderungen in der Netzhaut, besonders uber Periphlebitis retinalis bei Tuberkulosen. Klin Monatsbl Augenheilkd 49:28–34
6. Fleischer B (1914) Die juvenile, periphlebitis retinae mit ihren folgeercheinungen-eine echte Gefasstuberkulose der Netzhaut. Klin Monatsbl Augenheilkd 52:769–790
7. Donahue HC (1967) Ophthalmologic experience in a tuberculosis sanatorium. Am J Ophthalmol 64(4):742–748
8. Gilbert W (1935) Ueber Periphlebitis und Endovaskulitis der Netzhautgefasse nebst bemerkungen uber sklerotische. Tuberkulose und septische Aderhauterkrankungen. Klin Monatsbl Augenheilkd 94:335–349
9. Fountain JA, Werner RB (1984) Tuberculous retinal vasculitis. Retina 4(1):48–50
10. Rosen PH, Spalton DJ, Graham EM (1990) Intraocular tuberculosis. Eye 4(3):486–492
11. Ballantyne AJ, Michaelson IC (1937) A case of perivasculitis retinae associated with symptoms of cerebral disease. Br J Ophthalmol 21(1):22–35
12. Meyer W (1939) Die histologie der Menschlichen und experimentellen Augentuberkulose mit besonderer Beruck sichtigung der tuberkulosen Netzhauterkrankungen. Albrecht v Graefes Arch Ophthalmol 141:408–499
13. Elliot AJ (1954) Recurrent intraocular hemorrhage in young adults (Eales's disease); a report of thirty-one cases. Trans Am Ophthalmol Soc 52:811–875
14. Gass JDM, Olson CL (1976) Sarcoidosis with optic nerve and retinal involvement. Arch Ophthalmol 94(6):945–950
15. Chan C, Wetzig RP, Palestine AG (1987) Immunohistopathology of ocular sarcoidosis. Arch Ophthalmol 105:1398–1402
16. Arnold AC, Pepose JS, Hepler RS et al. (1984) Retinal periphlebitis and retinitis in multiple sclerosis. 1. Pathologic characteristics. Ophthalmology 91(3):255–262
17. Lucarelli MJ, Pepose JS, Arnold AC et al. (1991) Immunopathologic features of retinal lesions in multiple sclerosis. Ophthalmology 98(11):1652–1656

18. Green WR, Kincaid MC, Michels RG et al. (1981) Pars planitis. Trans Ophthalmol Soc UK 101(Pt 3):361–367

19. Wetzig RP, Chan CC, Nussenblatt RB (1988) Clinical and immunopathological studies of pars planitis in a family. Br J Ophthalmol 72(1):5–10

20. Ortega-Larrocea G, Arellanes-Garcia L (1995) Pars planitis: epidemiology and clinical outcome in a large community hospital in Mexico City. Int Ophthalmol 19(2):117–120

21. Holland GN (1994) Standard diagnostic criteria for the acute retinal necrosis syndrome. Executive Committee of the American Uveitis Society. Am J Ophthalmol 117(5):663–667

22. Culbertson WW, Blumenkranz MS, Haines H et al. (1982) The acute retinal necrosis syndrome. Part 2: Histopathology and etiology. Ophthalmology 89(12):1317–1325

23. Croxatto JO, Rao NA, McLean IW et al. (1990) Atypical histopathologic features in sympathetic ophthalmia: a study of a hundred cases. Int Ophthalmol 4:129–135

24. Graham EM, Stanford MR, Sanders MD et al. (1989) A point prevalence study of 150 patients with idiopathic retinal vasculitis: 1. Diagnostic value of ophthalmological features. Br J Ophthalmol 73(9):714–721

25. Graham EM, Stanford MR, Shilling JS et al. (1987) Neovascularisation associated with posterior uveitis. Br J Ophthalmol 71(11):826–833

26. Bentley CR, Stanford MR, Shilling JS et al. (1993) Macular ischaemia in posterior uveitis. Eye 7(3):411–444

27. Palmer HE, Zaman AG, Edelsten CE et al. (1995) Systemic morbidity in patients with isolated idiopathic retinal vasculitis. Lancet 346(8973):505–506

28. International Study Group for Behçet's Disease (1990) Criteria for diagnosis of Behçet's disease. Lancet 335(8697):1078–1080

29. Shah SM, Howard RS, Sarkies NJ (1988) Tuberculosis presenting as retinal vasculitis. J R Soc Med 81(4):232–233

30. Rothova A (2000) Ocular involvement in sarcoidosis. Br J Ophthalmol 84(1):110–116

31. Nowinski TS (1998) Ocular manifestations of sarcoidosis. Curr Opin Ophthalmol 9(6):80–84

32. Smith JA, Foster CS (1996) Sarcoidosis and its ocular manifestations. Int Ophthalmol Clin 36:109–125

33. Graham EM, Francis DA, Sanders MD et al. (1989) Ocular inflammatory changes in established multiple sclerosis. J Neurol Neurosurg Psychiatry 52(12):1360–1363

34. Engell T, Jensen OA, Klinken L (1985) Periphlebitis retinae in multiple sclerosis. A histopathological study of two cases. Acta Ophthalmol (Copenh) 63(1):83–88

35. Engell T, Andersen PK (1982) The frequency of periphlebitis retinae in multiple sclerosis. Acta Neurol Scand 65(6):601–608

36. Younge BR (1976) Fluorescein angiography and retinal venous sheathing in multiple sclerosis. Can J Ophthalmol 11(1):31–36

37. Malinowski SM (1993) Long-term visual outcome and complications associated with pars planitis. Ophthalmology 100:818–825

38. Chester GH, Blach RK, Cleary PE (1976) Inflammation in the region of the vitreous base. Pars planitis. Trans Ophthalmol Soc UK 96(1):151–157

39. Schmidt S, Wessels L, Augustin A et al. (2001) Patients with multiple sclerosis and concomitant uveitis/periphlebitis retinae are not distinct from those without intraocular inflammation. J Neurol Sci 187(1–2):49–53

40. Pepose JS, Holland GN, Nestor MS et al. (1985) Acquired immune deficiency syndrome. Pathogenic mechanism of ocular disease. Ophthalmology 92:472–484

41. Crouch ER, Goldberg MF (1975) Retinal periarteritis secondary to syphilis. Arch Ophthalmol 93:384–397

42. Halperin LS, Berger AS, Grand MG (1990) Syphilitic disc oedema and periphlebitis. Retina 10(3):223–225

43. Mendelsohn AD, Jampol LM (1984) Syphilitic retinitis. A cause of necrotizing retinitis. Retina 4(4):221–224

44. Morgan CM, Webb RM, O'Connor GR (1984) Atypical syphilitic chorioretinitis and vasculitis. Retina 4(4):225–231

Chapter 10

Masquerade Syndromes

10

Shouvik Saha, Elizabeth M. Graham

Core Messages

- Many neoplastic diseases may mimic intraocular inflammation
- Early diagnosis may result in sight- and life-prolonging intervention
- A high index of suspicion is crucial to diagnosing the underlying cause of intraocular inflammation in masquerade syndromes
- A neoplastic masquerade syndrome must be considered in any patient with a chronic uveitis

- without evidence of infection or other known cause of uveitis
- Many neoplastic masquerades may show an initial response to corticosteroids or immunosuppression
- Tissue biopsy with appropriate handling and laboratory analysis of specimens may be the key to diagnosis in many neoplastic masquerade syndromes

10.1 Introduction

The term "masquerade syndrome" was first used in 1967 to describe a case of conjunctival carcinoma that presented as chronic conjunctivitis [1]. Since then, the term has been applied to range of disorders that may present as intraocular inflammation. The disorders may be malignant or nonmalignant, but they share the common characteristic that intraocular inflammation is not due to an immune-mediated uveitides mechanism. Intraocular inflammation observed in a masquerade syndrome is secondary to another underlying disorder of the intraocular cells, and lesions are of a noninflammatory origin.

In a series of 828 consecutive uveitis patients seen in a tertiary centre, the prevalence of a masquerade syndrome was 5% ($n = 40$) [2]. These authors excluded bacterial and fungal endophthalmitis from their masquerade syndrome definition, although some investigators consider these to be masqueraders if running an indolent course. The diagnoses and their frequencies in this uveitis masquerade syndrome series are summarised in Table 10.1 [2]. This series reported a 2.3% frequency of malignant masquerade syndromes, with a time to diagnosis ranging from 1 to 48 months [2]. Early diagnosis of masquerading systemic disorders, especially malignancies, may allow for earlier intervention and hence improved sight and survival [3]. Thus, awareness, recognition and appropriate investigation of uveitic masquerade syndromes are of vital importance to the ophthalmologist. For the purposes of this uveitis update, neoplastic masquerade syndromes that may present as intraocular inflammation are discussed. The discussion is divided into lymphoproliferative and nonlymphoproliferative malignancies, but also mentions juvenile xanthogranuloma. Emphasis is placed on recognition and diagnosis of these entities rather than their management.

10.2 Lymphoproliferative Malignancies

Lymphoproliferative malignancies may simulate intraocular inflammation. Intraocular lymphomas can be divided into three main groups: primary intraocular lymphoma, primary uveal lymphoma and secondary intraocular lymphoma. Additionally, leukaemias and paraproteinaemias are briefly discussed.

10.2.1 Primary Intraocular Lymphoma

10.2.1.1 Introduction

Primary intraocular lymphoma (PIOL) is a subset of primary central nervous system lymphoma (PCNSL). PIOL involves retina, vitreous, or optic nerve head, with or without concomitant CNS involvement [4, 5]. It does not refer to a lymphoma arising outside CNS structures

10

Table 10.1. Masquerade syndrome diagnoses in a series with 828 uveitis patients [2]

Malignant (*n* = 19)	Nonmalignant (*n* = 21)
Lymphoma (*n* = 13)	Retinal detachment (*n* = 2)
Leukaemia (*n* = 3)	Diabetic retinopathy (*n* = 2)
Melanoma (*n* = 1)	Ocular ischaemic syndrome (*n* = 2)
Metastatic carcinoma (*n* = 1)	Hypertension (*n* = 2)
Retinoblastoma (*n* = 1)	Vitreous degeneration (*n* = 2)
	Dominant cystoid macular degeneration (*n* = 1)
	Hyperhomocystinaemia (*n* = 1)
	Hereditary Leber's optic atrophy (*n* = 1)
	Tapetoretinal degeneration (*n* = 1)
	Fundus flavimaculatus and intraocular foreign body (*n* = 1)
	Iris retraction syndrome (*n* = 1)
	Radiation retinopathy (*n* = 1)
	Branch retinal vein occlusion (*n* = 1)
	Retinal vessel occlusion (*n* = 1)
	Coats' disease (*n* = 1)

that metastasizes to the CNS or eye, in which case the uvea is mainly infiltrated (secondary intraocular lymphoma) [6]. The vast majority of PCNSL and PIOL is diffuse non-Hodgkin's B-cell lymphoma; however, T-cell lymphomas have been reported rarely [7, 8]. PCNSL has been referred to in the older literature by a number of terms, including reticulum cell sarcoma, microglioma, perithelial sarcoma and lymphosarcoma [3]. PCNSL has replaced these older terms based on progress in immunophenotyping techniques.

10.2.1.2 Epidemiology

PIOL is a rare malignancy. It is estimated to represent 1% of non-Hodgkin's lymphomas, 1% of intracranial tumours, and less than 1% of intraocular tumours [9]. PCNSL accounts for between 4 and 6% of primary brain tumours and 1–2% of extranodal lymphomas [10]. The exact incidence of PIOL is unknown [5]. However, the incidence of PCNSL has tripled from 0.027/100,000 in 1973 to 1/100,000 in the early 1990s, and it is inferred that a similar rise in PIOL has taken place [5, 11, 12]. The increased incidence of PCNSL has occurred in both the immunocompromised and immunocompetent. While the increases amongst the immunocompromised have been attributed to the wider use of immunosuppressive medications and HIV, the rise amongst the immunocompetent is unexplained [13].

The age of onset is usually during the sixth and seventh decades. However, any age may be affected, with the youngest reported patient being a three-year-old boy [14]. Opinion is divided regarding whether one gender is more commonly affected [6, 8]. There is no racial predilection [6].

10.2.1.3 Clinical Features

Both ocular and CNS features may present alone or together in PIOL. The eye is involved before the CNS in 50–80% of cases [6]. 60–80% of cases with a purely ocular presentation develop CNS disease within a mean of 29 months [15–17]. 50% of patients with PCNSL have multifocal disease at the time of presentation, with ocular involvement found in 15–25% [12, 18, 19]. Although most PIOL cases are initially unilateral, 75–80% eventually involve the other eye [5, 6].

In PIOL, the lymphoma cells are assumed to arise from and enter the eye through the blood stream. PIOL's most common masquerade presentation is of a chronic posterior uveitis. The most common symptoms are painless decrease in vision and floaters [2, 8, 14, 16]. Less common complaints include a red photophobic eye and ocular pain [20–22]. Visual acuity is usually dependent on the degree of vitritis, unless a coexistent optic neuropathy is present or lymphomatous deposits have involved the fovea. Macula oedema is rare. Even in the absence of an optic neuropathy, both colour vision and visual field may be reduced due to infiltration of the retina [23].

The frequency of anterior segment involvement reported in the literature varies. Slit lamp findings of mild anterior inflammation with cells, flare and keratitic precipitates are reported to be uncommon by Choi et al. [6], whereas others report between 50 and 75% of patients with anterior chamber cells at presentation [5, 8, 9, 24]. Pseudohypopyon has been reported [25]. Iris or angle neovascularisation with secondary glaucoma has been described [6]. PIOL has also been reported as a mass found in the iris or angle [24] (Fig. 10.1).

The most common and consistent ocular finding is hazy vitritis with clumps or sheets of vitreous cells being

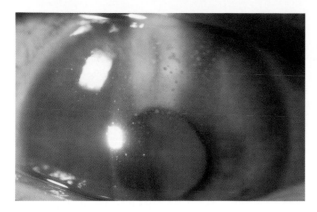

Fig. 10.1 Severe anterior uveitis with massive keratic precipitates all over the cornea and obvious tumour in the superior iris in a patient with recurrence of intraocular lymphoma

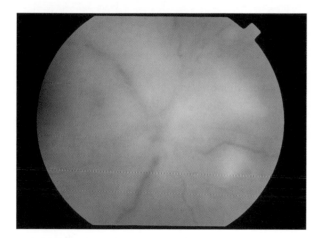

Fig. 10.2 Typical fundus changes in advanced intraocular lymphoma. The view is hazy because of the intense vitritis, but it is possible to see large pale areas of subretinal infiltrates and a hint of arteriolar sheathing

Table 10.2. Frequency of CNS features in PCNSL/PIOL at presentation [3]

General	Focal
Behavioural changes (24–73%)	Hemiparesis (40–50%)
	Cerebellar signs (15–40%)
Raised intracranial pressure (15–60%)	Seizures (2–33%)
	Cranial nerve palsies (5–31%)

lesions that have been mistaken for acute retinal necrosis and toxoplasmosis [3, 28]. Fundus appearances have masqueraded as frosted branch angiitis, exudative retinal detachments, nonpigmented choroidal melanoma, branch retinal artery occlusion with coexistent multifocal chorioretinal scars and retinal vasculitis [6, 29–32]. Infiltration of the optic nerve will produce signs of an optic neuropathy and may occasionally mimic a demyelinating optic neuritis [6].

CNS symptoms and signs may present at any time before or during the course of intraocular disease. Patients may present with general or focal neurological features. CNS lesions are most commonly found in the periventricular regions, and as a result the most common presenting features of PCNSL are personality alterations and changes in alertness. The frequency of CNS symptoms and signs at presentation in PCNSL/PIOL is detailed in Table 10.2 [3]. Seizures of new onset are a strong predictor of CNS involvement in PIOL [21]. 1–2% of PCNSL cases arise in the spinal cord [3]. However, no focal features such as radiculopathies have been reported in relation to spinal cord tumour involvement. In spite of this, lymphoma cells are found in the cerebrospinal fluid (CSF) of 42% of PCNSL patients [33].

PIOL most commonly masquerades as a chronic uveitis and is often treated initially with corticosteroids. The masquerade continues as initially there is a decrease in intraocular cells in response to corticosteroid therapy, as the majority of vitreous cells in PIOL are reactive, not malignant, and corticosteroids can be cytolytic to CNS lymphoma cells [6, 16]. The response does not last and eventually the uveitis becomes resistant to corticosteroids and the disease often progresses to involve the CNS. Initial inappropriate treatment with corticosteroids and immunosuppressives may contribute to low diagnostic yield from attempts at tissue biopsy such as vitrectomy [16, 20].

10.2.1.4 Fluorescein Angiography

The most common findings with fluorescein angiography relate to RPE disturbances and are largely nonspecific. Cassoux et al., in a series of 44 patients with ocular and

characteristic [5, 6, 8, 16, 26, 27]. Fundus appearances typically demonstrate scattered retinal white lesions and yellowish subretinal infiltrates or yellowish sub-retinal pigment epithelium (RPE) infiltrates [6] (Fig. 10.2). These are deposits of malignant cells [27]. They may be mistaken for white dot syndrome [6]. The sub-RPE deposits may enlarge and coalesce, resulting in detachments of the overlying RPE. The "leopard skin" pattern produced is considered pathognomonic by some authors, although it is not always present [6]. Sub-RPE lesions have been known to resolve spontaneously. If this spontaneous resolution occurs, the appearance of the fundus, with its multifocal small scars, may resemble ocular histoplasmosis syndrome [6].

Atypical fundus appearances have been reported. Extension through the RPE can produce discrete white

10

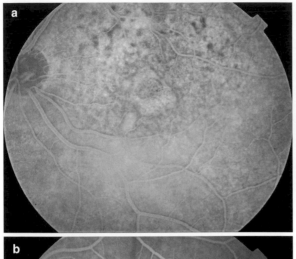

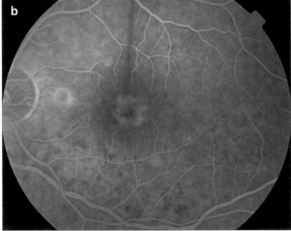

Fig. 10.3 In patients with subtle fundal changes, fluorescein angiography can be very useful. It can demonstrate abnormal retinal pigment epithelium and deep leakage into the fovea (**a**) and (**b**). Infiltration of the retinal pigment epithelium may give a leopard spot appearance, as shown in the superior part of this fundus (**c**)

CNS lymphoma, reported punctate hyperfluorescent lesions in 55%, round hypofluorescent lesions in 34%, vasculitis in 14%, papilloedema in 4% and cystoid macular oedema in 3% [34]. Velez et al., in a 17 patient series, reported their most common findings as granularity in 61%, RPE blockage in 55% and late staining in 45% [22]. The "leopard skin" pattern can look faint on fundoscopy but is highlighted on fluorescein angiography (Fig. 10.3). They found that these changes correlated well with histopathological findings of lymphoma cells between the RPE and Bruch's membrane. Less commonly found were pigment epithelial detachments and punctate hyperfluorescent lesions. Perivascular staining or leakage and cystoid macular oedema were rare in eyes without prior diagnostic surgical interventions. They noted that clinical

examination in some cases did not correlate well with fluorescein angiography.

10.2.1.5   Ultrasonography

Ophthalmic ultrasound may be useful for narrowing the diagnosis, but findings are nonspecific [3, 5]. Ursea et al. reported a 13-patient PCNSL/PIOL series, all of whom had abnormal ultrasonography [35]. The most common findings reported are vitreous debris (77%), choroidal–scleral thickening (46%) and widening of the optic nerve (31%) [36]. Elevated chorioretinal lesions were reported in 23% of cases and retinal detachments in 15% [37].

10.2.2   Special Investigations

Given the nonspecificity of ophthalmic findings in PIOL, it is important to undertake a thorough general medical and neurological assessment, including chest radiograph, blood tests and other general investigations to screen for systemic illness and exclude specific causes of uveitis before embarking on special investigations.

10.2.2.1   Neuroradiology

Neuroradiological investigations are mandatory in cases of suspected PIOL due to the high risk of CNS involvement. Radiological features of PCNSL vary between the immunocompetent and immunocompromised.

In the immunocompetent, CT typically shows multiple, diffuse, periventricular, iso or hyperdense lesions before contrast. After contrast injection, dense periventricular enhancement appears and may involve the corpus callosum. Systemic corticosteroid therapy may alter this appearance, with resolution of the periventricular enhancement [3]. When PCNSL recurs, lesions may appear different, with solid ring-like enhancement away from the ventricles [3]. Magnetic resonance imaging (MRI) typically shows hypointense lesions on T1 weighting and hyperintense lesions on T2 weighting [18]. At diagnosis, neuroradiological lesions are single in up to 70% of cases but are usually multifocal in later stages [5].

In AIDS-related PCNSL, CT findings typically show irregular, ring-like enhancement in the basal ganglia, with surrounding oedema and mass effect. This is radiologically indistinguishable from cerebral toxoplasmosis. Necrosis and haemorrhages are also common. MRI in these patients may show diffuse disease involving the deep grey matter nuclei and white matter tracts rather than a mass. T2-weighted images show extensive hyperintensities in the pons, cerebellum, white matter and basal ganglia.

10.2.2.2 Cerebrospinal Fluid Analysis

CSF from lumbar puncture may lead to a diagnosis of PIOL and obviate the need for the higher morbidity procedure of vitreous biopsy. Lymphoma cells have been identified in the CSF of 25% of patients with known MRI lesions [36]. If lymphoma cells are found in the CSF, then no other diagnostic procedures are necessary to achieve a tissue diagnosis. Some authors argue that CSF specimens contain less necrotic debris than vitreous sampling and lymphoma cells may be easier to recognize on conventional cytology [16]. However, this should be balanced against lumbar puncture yielding fewer cells than vitreous sampling techniques for immunophenotyping studies [3]. Overall, consensus opinion recommends lumbar puncture as the first step in reaching a tissue diagnosis [3, 5].

10.2.3 Tissue Biopsy

Given the often nonspecific clinical and general investigative findings, tissue analysis is fundamental in establishing a diagnosis of PIOL.

10.2.3.1 Vitreous Sampling

Vitreous sampling is commonly used to obtain tissue for analysis. However, nondiagnostic sampling may result for a number of reasons. Vitreous samples are typically less cellular than the clinical appearance would suggest [9]. Many of the lymphocytes present in vitreous may be inflammatory, not neoplastic [9]. Previous corticosteroid therapy has been reported to be cytolytic to lymphoma cells and decrease the viability of lymphoma cells obtained in samples, further reducing the diagnostic yield [16]. Multiple vitreous samples may be required before a diagnosis is made [6, 9, 16].

The two techniques for vitreous sampling are fine needle aspiration (FNA) and pars plana vitrectomy (PPV). The sample size is limited in FNA; however, the technique results in less mechanical disruption to cell structures [19]. Bardestein reported the technique to be diagnostic in several cases previously hampered by mechanical vitrector artifacts [9]. FNA can be performed safely and effectively in the outpatient setting [37]. In a series of 26 patients with presumed PIOL, FNA alone was able to confirm or exclude the diagnosis in all but two patients, and both of these patients had prior treatment with corticosteroids [37]. PPV is more widely used than FNA for vitreous sampling. Despite a more invasive surgical approach than FNA, PPV affords a number of advantages. PPV may have a therapeutic effect in clearing vitreous opacity in the symptomatic patient [9]. Also, PPV yields a larger vitre-

ous sample for analysis. This may help compensate for low cellular concentration due to prior corticosteroid therapy, vitrector mechanical disruption and the presence of reactive lymphocytes [6, 9].

Appropriate handling of the vitreous specimen after sampling is crucial to diagnostic analysis. The specimen must be transported to the laboratory as quickly as possible, as lymphoma cells undergo morphological degradation within 60 min [38]. However, this should also be done as gently as possible to minimise mechanical disruption to the fragile cells [38]. Whitcup et al. also suggested discontinuing corticosteroids prior to vitrectomy and using cell culture media for storage instead of saline to improve the diagnostic yield of vitrectomy specimens [39].

10.2.3.2 Other Tissue Sampling Techniques

Retinal or chorioretinal sampling may be considered if vitreous samples are nondiagnostic. Several techniques for the subretinal aspiration of neoplastic lymphocytes deposited between the RPE and Bruch's membrane have been described [19, 30, 40]. Subretinal aspiration preserves anatomic boundaries to contain the tumour and causes minimal tissue disruption [6]. Another technique is retinal or chorioretinal biopsy, which excises a segment of diffuse retinal or subretinal infiltrate [6]. A trans-scleral approach to the sub-RPE space has been described, although this is more invasive than trans-retinal approaches [41]. Other means of acquiring tissue for diagnosis that are rarely reported include anterior chamber paracentesis, iris biopsy or diagnostic enucleation if vision has been lost [25, 38].

10.2.4 Tissue Analysis Techniques

10.2.4.1 Cytology

Cytology is the gold standard for diagnosis of PIOL [19]. Abnormal lymphoid cells have several cytological characteristics. They are usually large, pleomorphic cells with high nuclear/cytoplasmic ratios, irregular nuclear outlines, prominent nucleoli or chromocentres, occasional mitotic figures and coarse chromatin patterns [42, 43]. However, even with rapid and gentle transport to the laboratory, specimen analysis can be difficult. In spite of centrifuging to increase the concentration of them, few characteristic lymphoma cells are usually present in vitreous specimens. Most vitreous samples have a heavy content of reactive lymphocytes, histiocytes, necrotic debris and fibrous material, obscuring lymphoma cell recognition even to an expert ophthalmic cytopathologist [16]. Although cytology is the accepted gold standard for diagnosis of PIOL, a false-negative rate of up to 30% has been reported in the literature [44]. It is thus recognized other tissue analysis techniques have an adjunctive role in the diagnosis of PIOL.

10.2.4.2 Immunohistochemistry

Categorization of vitreous cells by their cell-surface markers provides useful supplementary information in the diagnosis of PIOL [19]. Davis et al. have reported some cases in which cell-surface markers remain detectable even if the cytological preservation of cells is inadequate to reach a diagnosis on morphology alone [45].

Immunohistochemistry can be performed by either the microscopic examination of slides of properly stained cells or by flow cytometry. Both techniques have been used for the diagnosis of PIOL [19]. Both techniques rely on antibodies binding to specific antigens of interest on the cell surface. A "panel" of antibodies is selected based on the probable diagnosis and the number of cells that are available for labelling. Table 10.3 shows common cell surface markers used in the analysis of vitreous cells [19]. PIOL is typically a large B-cell lymphoma, and antibody selection concentrates on B-cell markers. Cell surface markers CD19 and CD20 are pan B-cell proteins that are highly expressed in B-cell lymphomas [6]. CD22 is found on early B-cells, and its presence is suggestive of B-cell lymphoma [6]. The kappa and lambda light-chain immunoglobulins are additional markers [6]. A significant preponderance of one type of light chain over another suggests B-cell lymphoma [19]. Immunohistochemistry has also been used to demonstrate BCL-2, BCL-6 and MUM1 on B-cell PIOL cells [46]. BCL-2 has an antiapoptotic function and is overexpressed following the translocation t(14:18). This places the BCL2 gene under the control of the IgH promoter. BCL-6 is a B-cell marker that is normally inactivated as B cells move from the germinal centre into the marginal zone during B-cell differentiation. MUM1 is a protein involved in the control of plasma cell differentiation [5]. Concomitant expression of BCL-6 and MUM1 has been shown in systemic diffuse large B-cell lymphoma [5]. A similar pattern of expression has been demonstrated in a series of five patients with PIOL

Table 10.3. Common cell surface markers used in the analysis of vitreous cells [19]

Markers	Specificity	Interpretation
T-cell markers		
CD2, CD3, CD5, CD7	Pan T-cell	High expression in active uveitis or T-cell lymphomas. Aberrant expression of some of the "pan" markers but not others increases suspicion of lymphoma.
CD4	T-helper	Increased relative to CD8 in active uveitis; mycosis fungoides.
CD8	T-suppressor	Increased relative to CD4 in inactive uveitis; mycosis fungoides with shift in immunophenotype.
B-cell markers		
CD19, CD20	Pan B-cell	High expression in B-cell lymphomas. Increased in inactive uveitis relative to active uveitis.
CD22	Early B-cell	Supportive of B-cell lymphoma, but can also present on normal cells.
Kappa: Lambda	Light-chain immunoglobulin	Heterogeneous populations of B-cells have roughly equal proportions of kappa and lambda light-chain immunoglobulins. B-cell lymphomas usually have a K:L or L:K ratio of >3. Lack of kappa or lambda expression in a predominantly B-cell population is suggestive of lymphoma.
Activation markers		
HLA-DR	MHC class II	Immunologically active cells consistent with inflammation.
CD25	IL-2 receptor	Immunologically active cells consistent with inflammation. Expressed on activated T and B lymphocytes.
Other cell lineages		
CD14	Monocyte/ macrophage	May be increased in infections. Consistent with a heterogeneous inflammatory response.
CD56	Natural killer cells	May be increased in infections. Consistent with a heterogeneous inflammatory response.
CD33	Pan myeloid	Neutrophils, eosinophils, basophils. May be increased in infections. Consistent with a heterogeneous inflammatory response.

[47]. T-cell lymphoma markers often used include CD3, CD4 and CD8. However, these may be elevated in active uveitis as well as T-cell lymphoma [6].

Flow cytometry allows up to three or four different monoclonal antibodies to be applied to an aliquot of suspected lymphoma cells, as opposed to slide-based techniques in which a separate slide is required for each cell-surface marker [42]. This allows for a larger detection panel of antibodies to be used per vitreous specimen, improving the detection of T-cell lymphomas [19]. An algorithm of cell-surface marker testing based on the number of cells available for staining in flow cytometry has been developed by Wilson et al. to maximise the probability of detecting B-cell lymphomas [47].

10.2.4.3 Cytokines

Vitreal levels of interleukins IL-10, IL-6 and IL-12 measured by enzyme-linked immunosorbent assay (ELISA) have been proposed as an ancillary test in the diagnosis of PIOL. IL-10 appears to be preferentially secreted by malignant B-cells [19], whereas IL-6 and IL-12 are thought be produced more by inflammatory cells. The use of IL-10:IL-6 or IL-10:IL-12 ratios, despite biological plausibility, has been controversial, with conflicting evidence from small studies [48, 49]. Elevated vitreal levels of IL-10 are considered suggestive but not diagnostic of B-cell lymphoma.

10.2.4.4 Molecular Analysis

Molecular techniques that were developed to improve the diagnosis of systemic lymphoma may have an adjunctive role in the diagnosis of PIOL [19]. Microdissection to isolate abnormal cells or laser-capture microscopy can be used to increase the diagnostic yield for molecular analysis. Isolated suspicious cells are then examined by polymerase chain reaction (PCR) [50]. Monoclonality in a B-cell population can be demonstrated by PCR for heavy-chain immunoglobulin (IgH) gene rearrangements. In a survey of microdissected atypical lymphoid cells from 50 cases of PIOL, Chan et al. demonstrated that 100% showed monoclonality with IgH gene rearrangements using PCR for the third hypervariable or complementarity-determining region (CDR3) [51]. PCR is not always effective. In a series of 36 patients with PIOL, Merle-Beral et al. found seven in whom IgH gene rearrangements could not be demonstrated. They attributed this to somatic hypermutation preventing annealing of primers [38]. PCR has been used to detect gene rearrangements for the t(14:18)

translocations at the major breakpoint region (mbr) and minor cluster region (mcr) of the bcl-2 protein in vitreous specimen lymphoma cells [5, 50, 51]. Rearrangement of the T-cell receptor gamma gene holds promise as a diagnostic technique for intraocular T-cell lymphomas [19, 52].

10.2.5 Treatment

The optimal treatment for PIOL has not yet been defined. Therapy for PCNSL may not be directly applicable to PIOL.

10.2.5.1 Radiation Therapy

Radiation therapy was historically considered a first-line treatment. Despite early remission with dramatic resolution of symptoms and signs, nearly all patients developed early CNS progression and died, with a two-year survival rate of less than 20% reported [53]. Radiation therapy cannot be repeated if the patient relapses. Neurotoxicity has been a significant problem, especially in elderly patients [54]. Radiotherapy-associated ocular complications have been reported in several series [55]. These problems have led to an emphasis on chemotherapy [55], although ocular radiotherapy is beneficial in severely ill patients with a poor general prognosis.

10.2.5.2 Chemotherapy

The major hurdle with chemotherapy for PIOL has been the blood–ocular barrier, which prevents therapeutic drug concentrations being reached intraocularly. Methotrexate (MTX) and cytosine arabinoside (Ara-C) feature at the forefront of most chemotherapy regimens on account of their ability to penetrate the blood–ocular barrier [5].

Intravenous high-dose MTX and high-dose Ara-C have both been used alone or in combination with other chemotherapeutic agents with reasonable success [5]. Intrathecal MTX has been shown to have some effect in the treatment of PIOL [56, 57]. Intravitreal MTX has been used to treat both isolated and recurrent ocular lymphoma [58]. Intravitreal MTX, unfortunately, does not treat CNS disease. Chemotherapy followed by autologous stem-cell transplantation has been tried with some success, suggesting that this technique may be useful in refractory or recurrent cases [59]. Trofosamide, an alkylating cytostatic agent commonly used as maintenance therapy for haematological malignancies, has been used orally as an alternative to conventional treatments with good results, albeit in a study of two patients [60].

10

10.2.5.3 Combination Chemotherapy and Radiotherapy

The current consensus on treating PIOL with concurrent CNS disease is systemic high-dose MTX-based chemotherapy with radiotherapy to the globes [5]. Isolated eye disease should be treated similarly, although radiotherapy complications and promising results from high-dose MTX regimens may indicate a solely chemotherapeutic MTX-based strategy to be a superior choice [5]. Recurrence of intraocular lymphoma alone should be treated with intravitreal MTX. Further studies are essential to determine optimal treatment strategies and investigate new chemotherapeutic agents, but are difficult to perform given the rarity of these malignancies.

10.2.6 Prognosis

PIOL remains an ominous diagnosis. Most patients with PIOL will progress to CNS involvement within two years. However, newer treatments have improved median survival from 12–18 months to more than three years [6].

Summary for the Clinician

- PIOL involves retina, vitreous, or optic nerve head, with or without concomitant CNS involvement
- PIOL most commonly masquerades as a chronic posterior uveitis; hints on presentation are reduced colour vision, visual field and absence of cystoid macular oedema
- Initial inappropriate treatment with corticosteroids and immunosuppressives may contribute to low diagnostic yield from attempts at tissue biopsy such as vitrectomy
- CSF from lumbar puncture may lead to a diagnosis of PIOL and obviate the need for the higher morbidity procedure of vitreous biopsy
- Vitreous sampling is commonly used to obtain tissue for analysis; however, nondiagnostic sampling is common
- Appropriate handling of the vitreous specimen after sampling is crucial to diagnostic analysis
- Although cytology is the accepted gold standard for diagnosis of PIOL, a false-negative rate of up to 30% has been reported
- Immunohistochemistry, vitreal cytokine levels and molecular analysis are useful adjunctive diagnostic techniques

---

10.2.7 Primary Uveal Lymphoma

The primary uveal lymphomas are the least common of the intraocular lymphomas. Less than seventy cases have been reported in the literature. As primary uveal lymphomas are generally clinically indolent, they have previously been misnamed "reactive lymphoid hyperplasia" and "uveal pseudotumours". However, the demonstration of monoclonality amongst infiltrating lymphocyte populations and immunophenotyping led to their redefinition as low-grade B-cell NHL [61, 62]. Most recently, Coupland et al. proposed their subtyping as extranodal marginal zone B-cell lymphomas of MALT type according to the REAL lymphoma classification [63] on the basis of their morphological, immunophenotypical and clinical similarities [64].

The typical patient is a man in the fifth decade, although the reported range varies from 30 to 81 years [3]. Presenting symptoms include recurrent episodes of blurred vision, gradual painless loss of vision and metamorphopsia [65]. Most are unilateral [65]. Anterior uveitis with pain, redness, photophobia, keratitic precipitates and hypopyon have been described [3] (Fig. 10.4a). A vitritis is often absent or sparse in contrast to PIOL. Examination in the early stages may show multifocal, creamy choroidal lesions which may simulate inflammatory uveitides such as birdshot choroidopathy or sarcoidosis [3] (Fig. 10.4b). Cystoid macular oedema may be present [3]. Later manifestations include serous retinal detachments and diffuse choroidal thickening [3]. Fundus lesions evolve slowly and can remain stable in size and appearance over a number of years [3]. Raised intraocular pressure and glaucoma are common. This can arise from increased episcleral venous pressure or from angle closure. Angle closure may be secondary to rubeosis iridis, anterior synechiae or anterior movement of the iris–lens diaphragm [3]. Lymphocytic infiltration of angle structures and Schlemm's canal is a common finding, and has been suggested as a mechanism for open-angle glaucoma in these patients [66]. In advanced cases, subconjunctival or episcleral extension can develop [65] (Fig. 10.4c). These may appear as a pink discoloration and thickening of the episclera or conjunctiva, and it is said that—unlike conjunctival lymphomas—they are not freely movable [3]. There may be an initial response to corticosteroid therapy [65].

In contrast to PIOL, ultrasonography is an extremely useful diagnostic procedure. On ultrasonography, the choroid is diffusely thickened with low reflectivity and lacks choroidal or scleral excavation [3]. Common differential diagnoses considered include posterior scleritis,

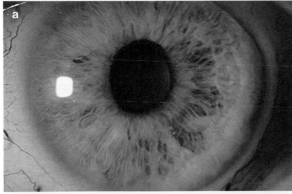

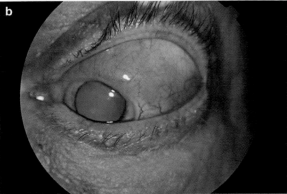

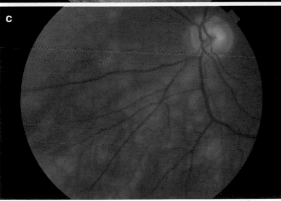

Fig. 10.4 An elderly gentleman presents with a chronic uveitis with granulomatous keratic precipitates (**a**), which persist despite treatment for three years. He then develops a large fleshy lesion in the superior conjunctiva (**b**) and is also found to have retinal pigment epithelial disease (**c**). Biopsy of the conjunctival lesion showed MALToma

performed. In the majority of primary uveal lymphoma cases the eyes have been ultimately enucleated due to pain from glaucoma or because of difficulties in clinically differentiating the uveal changes from a malignant uveal melanoma [65]. Tissue biopsy techniques reported in the literature include biopsy of episcleral tumour nodules, chorioretinal biopsy and fine-needle aspiration biopsy [65].

On microscopy, primary uveal lymphomas consist of a dense infiltration of small tumour cells with occasional blasts in the marginal zone surrounding reactive follicles [65]. Morphological features such as "follicular colonisation" and "lymphoepithelial lesions" may be present [65]. These provide supporting evidence for the neoplastic nature of these lesions [63]. Immunohistochemical studies show a B-cell dominance of the infiltrating lymphocytes, often with an aberrant expression of the T-cell antigen CD43 as well as monotypical expression of an immunoglobulin light chain and or heavy chain [64]. The degree of plasmacellular differentiation can be extensive in primary uveal lymphoma [62, 64, 66]. Neoplastic plasmacytoid cells usually demonstrate a loss of plasma-cell-related antigens compared with reactive plasma cells [64]. The monoclonality of the B-cell population can be demonstrated using IgH-PCR [65], supporting the neoplastic basis of this entity.

Low-dose irradiation is considered the treatment of choice, although resolution has been achieved with moderately high doses of systemic corticosteroids [65]. The prognosis for primary uveal lymphoma is very good, with only exceptional cases of dissemination or CNS involvement [67].

> ## Summary for the Clinician
>
> - Primary uveal lymphomas are the least common of the intraocular lymphomas
> - Common differential diagnoses considered include posterior scleritis, uveal effusion syndrome and diffuse uveal melanoma, and ultrasound may help differentiate these
> - The prognosis for primary uveal lymphoma is very good, with only exceptional cases of dissemination or CNS involvement

uveal effusion syndrome and diffuse uveal melanoma [3]. Several ultrasonographic features may help distinguish these. Posterior scleritis has high reflectivity from scleral thickening [3]. Uveal effusion syndrome does not present with extrascleral lesions, and diffuse uveal melanomas tend to have less-extensive choroidal thickening [3].

Clinical and ultrasonographic features alone are not specific enough for diagnosis and tissue analysis must be

10.2.8 Secondary Intraocular Lymphomas

Secondary intraocular lymphomas are systemic lymphomas that have metastasized to structures within the eye. Secondary intraocular lymphomas tend to involve the uveal tract, in contrast to PIOL. Predominantly retinal disease without uveal infiltration is rare but has been reported [68]. Secondary intraocular lymphomas are invariably of non-Hodgkin's type, with Hodgkin's lymphoma presenting intraocularly being exceptional [69, 70]. In patients with secondary intraocular lymphomas, systemic findings usually precede ocular findings, with most patients having a known history of systemic lymphoma [71], although ocular disease may be the presenting sign of systemic lymphoma [72]. Treatment is dependent on the extent of the disease, type of lymphoma and comorbidities [67]. In patients with systemic NHL, the extent of intraocular involvement and visual loss tends to parallel the severity of systemic disease [71]. The long-term prognosis in patients with intraocular involvement from systemic NHL is poor [71]. The mean interval from ocular diagnosis to death is 31 months [71].

10.2.8.1   Diffuse Large B-Cell Lymphoma

The most common systemic lymphoma subtype to affect the eye is diffuse large B-cell lymphoma (DLBCL) [67]. Conjunctival or orbital involvement is relatively common but intraocular involvement is rare [3]. In the posterior segment, signs may include a solitary choroidal mass with adjacent exudative retinal detachment, vitritis, retinal vasculitis, necrotizing retinitis and diffuse choroiditis or focal uveal masses [3]. In the anterior segment, granulomatous anterior uveitis with hypopyon has been reported [72]. In general, systemic NHL involving the eye tends to involve the uveal tract, whereas patients with PIOL have vitreous, retinal or sub-RPE involvement. However, patients with advanced disease are most likely to present with overlapping features [68]. Diagnostic approaches include vitrectomy, vitreoretinal biopsy, fine-needle aspiration biopsy, transscleral choroidal biopsy, and diagnostic enucleation [68, 71].

Morphologically, it may be difficult to determine whether ocular DLBCL represents a primary or secondary intraocular lymphoma [67]. Although retinal infiltration usually suggests PIOL, there may be exceptions [67]. Coupland et al. have demonstrated that the expression of various immunoglobulin transcription factors in systemic DLBCL is different from those of PIOL/PCNSL [73]. Clonal analysis with PCR may help differentiate between clonal proliferations arising from the same tumour and two distinct primary lymphomas [67].

10.2.8.2   Intravascular B-Cell Lymphoma (Malignant Angioendotheliomatosis)

Intravascular B-cell lymphoma is a rare subtype of diffuse large B-cell lymphoma, characterized by the presence of tumour cells in the blood vessels, especially capillaries [74]. Clinically, dermatological and neurological mani-

festations dominate but ophthalmic involvement is frequent [75]. Ocular findings reported include visual loss, vitreous cells, retinal artery occlusion, retinal vascular and pigment epithelial alterations, choroidal infarction, exudative retinal detachment, nystagmus and cortical blindness [74, 75]. Diagnosis has been reported from enucleation and necropsy [74, 75]. Intravascular B-cell lymphoma is a high-grade lymphoma with a grave prognosis that responds poorly to chemotherapy [74].

10.2.8.3   T or T/Nk-Cell Lymphomas

Close to 50 cases of intraocular manifestations of T-cell lymphomas have been published in the literature [76]. Approximately 80% of these patients had a primary tumour located extraocularly; of these, one-third were diagnosed with mycosis fungoides and approximately one-half with systemic (non-mycosis) lymphoma [76]. Of the rest, patients appeared to have PCNSL/PIOL of T-cell origin [76]. All these lymphoma entities are very aggressive, and patients usually die soon after initial diagnosis [67].

In the majority of case reports involving systemic T-cell lymphomas, patients present primarily with anterior segment involvement mimicking an anterior uveitis [3]. This has been reported to progress to pseudohypopyon in some cases [25, 77]. Secondary glaucoma is a common finding with uveal involvement, probably due to direct tumour infiltration of the angle or secondary to angle neovascularisation [24]. Intraocular T-cell lymphoma has been reported as mimicking a ring melanoma [78]. In this case it was the first manifestation of systemic disease later found in the bone marrow [78]. Posterior segment involvement has also been described, with findings including opacities of the vitreous body, vitritis, chorioretinitis, subretinal infiltrates and retinal vasculitis [31, 79–81].

Mycosis fungoides, a cutaneous T-cell lymphoma, not uncommonly involves periocular tissues [3]. Intraocular extension of mycosis fungoides is rare [3]. Clinicopathological features observed include granulomatous anterior uveitis, posterior synechiae, dense vitreous opacities, large creamy-white retinal infiltrates, retinal haemorrhages and tumour infiltration of the vitreous, inner retina, optic nerve and choroid. Diagnosis is usually confirmed from enucleation or at necropsy [81–85]. Interestingly, Lois et al. have reported a case in which the vitreous infiltrate showed a different immunophenotypic dominance to the skin biopsy taken seven years earlier, and suggested that the immunophenotypic shift may have been related to the poor outcome [85]. All of the patients reported in the literature had a long history of mycosis fungoides at the time of onset of intraocular disease; the median duration being seven years [76]. Intraocular extension is a grave sign, with patients dying within weeks or months of ocular presentation [76].

Extranodal natural killer T-cell lymphoma (NKTL) is uncommon except in oriental, Native-American and Hispanic populations [81]. It is in the spectrum of disorders associated with Epstein–Barr virus infection [86]. The nasal cavity is the most common site of involvement, but histopathologically identical tumours may be found in a range of extranodal sites [86]. Nasal NKTL is best known for orbital infiltration, but a number of cases with signs of intraocular inflammation have been described [80, 81, 86, 87]. Anterior uveitis, vitritis, preretinal infiltrates, retinal and subretinal haemorrhages, rhegmatogenous retinal detachment and macular hole have been reported in association with NKTL [80, 81, 86, 87]. Importantly, signs of intraocular inflammation may precede the diagnosis of NKTL [81]. Generally, the prognosis is grave [81].

Adult T-cell leukaemia/lymphoma (ATLL) is characterized by an extremely aggressive clinical course, leukaemic or lymphomatous proliferation of hyperlobulated peripheral T-cells, and an association with infection by the retrovirus human T-lymphotropic virus type I (HTLV-1) [88]. Intraocular lesions in ATLL may mimic intraocular inflammation. Retinal infiltrates, subretinal infiltrates, and a masquerade presentation as acute retinal necrosis or herpetic retinitis have been described [88, 89]. Diagnosis has been established by vitrectomy, chorioretinal biopsy or at post mortem examination [88–90].

> **Summary for the Clinician**
>
> ■ Secondary intraocular lymphomas tend to involve the uveal tract, in contrast to PIOL
> ■ Systemic findings usually precede ocular findings, with most patients having a known history of systemic lymphoma, although ocular disease may be the presenting sign of systemic lymphoma
> ■ In patients with systemic NHL, the extent of intraocular involvement and visual loss tends to parallel the severity of systemic disease
> ■ The long-term prognosis is poor

10.2.9 Leukaemias

It is estimated that leukaemic involvement of the eye occurs in up to 90% of cases and eye symptoms are rarely the initial presentation of leukaemia [91]. The eye is involved, directly or indirectly, much more frequently in acute leukaemias than in chronic leukaemias [91]. Clinically, the retina shows leukaemic involvement more often than any other ocular tissue [91]. Retinal findings include intraretinal haemorrhages, cotton wool spots, Roth spots, microaneurysms and peripheral neovascularisation [3]. Occasionally, leukaemic cells can break through the internal limiting membrane into the vitreous cavity to simulate vitritis [3]. Bilateral vitritis was the ocular presentation in a case of large B-cell lymphoma transformation of chronic lymphocytic leukaemia (Richter's syndrome) [92]. When the choroid is infiltrated, exudative retinal detachments can occur [3]. Angiographically, this may mimic the typical pattern of Vogt–Koyanagi–Harada disease or posterior scleritis, demonstrating multiple, pinpoint serous detachments of the retina and RPE [3]. Other masquerade presentations include anterior uveitis, spontaneous hyphaema, heterochromia iridis or pseudohypopyon, which is typically grey-yellow in colour [3]. The presence of malignant leukaemic cells may be confirmed by vitrectomy or aspiration of anterior chamber pseudohypopyon [91] (Fig. 10.5). Secondary ocular manifestations may occur many years after initial diagnosis in chronic leukaemias [93].

> **Summary for the Clinician**
>
> ■ It is estimated that leukaemic involvement of the eye occurs in up to 90% of cases
> ■ Eye symptoms may be the initial presentation of leukaemia
> ■ Secondary ocular manifestations may occur many years after initial diagnosis in chronic leukaemias

10.2.10 Paraproteinaemias

Amongst the paraproteinaemias, only multiple myeloma has been reported to manifest features that could mimic intraocular inflammation. A few cases of myeloma patients with anterior chamber plasma cells and even pseudohypopyon have been described [94–96].

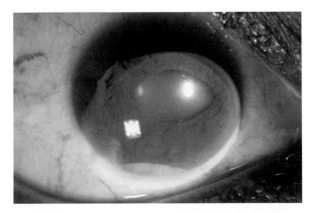

Fig. 10.5 A pseudohypopyon in a patient with a recurrence of acute lymphocytic leukaemia

10.3   Nonlymphoproliferative Malignancies

Nonlymphoproliferative malignancies may also simulate intraocular inflammation. Uveal melanoma, retinoblastoma and ocular metastases are discussed. Additionally, juvenile xanthogranuloma is described.

10.3.1   Uveal Melanoma

Ocular melanomas include lesions of the uvea, conjunctiva and eyelid. More than 85% of all ocular melanomas are uveal [97], and these are the tumours that most frequently masquerade as intraocular inflammation [98]. Malignant melanoma of the uveal tract is the most common primary intraocular tumour in adults [97]. The overall incidence is estimated at five per million per year [97]. The tumours are more common in older individuals and in Caucasians [97]. They are more common in those with blue or grey eyes [97]. There is no sex predominance [97]. Unlike cutaneous melanomas, they are rarely if ever caused by inherited mutations [99]. They can develop from melanocytoma or ocular melanocytosis [99]. The role of sunlight is controversial [99].

10.3.1.1   Clinical Features

Melanoma can present anywhere along the uveal tract. The most frequent site is the choroid (90%) [99]. The ciliary body and iris are less commonly involved; 5–10 and 3% respectively [99]. When the choroid is involved, 40% of tumours at presentation extend to within 3 mm of the optic disc or fovea [99].

45% of patients are asymptomatic at presentation, but conversely 21% of patients report that their tumour was not detected when they first presented [99]. Symptomatic patients may report flashing lights or scotomas [98]. If the macula is affected, the patient may describe metamorphopsia. An increase in hypermetropia or a decrease in myopia may be found [98]. When masquerading as intraocular inflammation, uveal melanoma may present as unilateral uveitis [98]. Iris lesions may produce anterior chamber cells and flare [98]. Ciliary body melanomas may produce dilated episcleral vessels, classically termed sentinel vessels [100]. The patients may receive a misdiagnosis of episcleritis or scleritis [100]. Secondary glaucoma, cataract and exudative retinal detachments are recognized features [99, 101]. Posterior melanomas are less commonly mistaken for intraocular inflammation, but can produce a focal choroidal mass that resembles a sarcoid or tuberculous granuloma or posterior scleritis [98].

Extraocular extension can occur along sclera channels for posterior ciliary arteries, vortex veins and drainage vessels [99]. Metastatic disease occurs by haematogenous spread and is invariably fatal within a year [99].

10.3.1.2   Diagnosis

The diagnostic accuracy of an experienced examiner for a typical uveal melanoma is excellent [102]. The most characteristic findings are development of a collar-button or mushroom-shaped configuration because of tumour rupture through Bruch's membrane [98]. Other features suggestive of melanoma include associated subretinal fluid and the presence of orange pigmentation, visualized because of the contrast between lipofuscin and melanin [98].

In the atypical masquerading case, diagnosis is more difficult and may be assisted by special investigations. Fluorescein angiography of choroidal tumours is widely performed, although it is recognized that indocyanine green angiography provides greater information about the tumour itself, also defining the tumour margins more clearly in some cases [99]. Ultrasonography is useful for measuring tumour dimensions and assessing response to treatments [103]. It is also useful for examining the posterior segment when the media are opaque, and can identify extraocular extension [103]. High-frequency ultrasound is valuable for iris and ciliary tumours [103]. The internal acoustic reflectivity may be useful in difficult diagnostic cases [103]. Other imaging modalities such as CT, MRI and CT/PET have been used for diagnostic purposes in uveal melanoma, but ultrasound is considered superior [103]. With some small lesions, the diagnosis may sometimes only be made during close progressive follow-up. Where diagnosis remains in doubt, fine-needle aspiration biopsy with appropriate immunohistochemical analysis may be considered [99]. It seems likely, with advances in cytogenetics, that biopsy will be used more widely to guide optimal management strategies [99].

10.3.1.3   Management

Treatment options for the primary tumour include brachytherapy, proton beam radiotherapy, transpupillary thermotherapy, trans-scleral local resection, endoresection and enucleation [99]. No single method has proved to be superior in preventing metastatic disease [104]. It appears that all methods of local treatment are associated with a similar prognosis [104]. Risk factors for metastatic disease include tumour dimensions, ciliary body involvement, cell type, extravascular matrix patterns and cytogenetics [99]. Abnormalities related to chromosomes 3, 6 and 8 are strongly related to tumour behaviour and survival probability [105]. Results of systemic treatments for metastatic uveal melanoma continue to be discouraging [104]. Overall, uveal melanoma related mortality is 30% by 5 years and 45% by 15 years [106].

Summary for the Clinician

■ More than 85% of all ocular melanomas are uveal, and these are the tumours that most frequently masquerade as intraocular inflammation

■ Risk factors for metastatic disease include tumour dimensions, ciliary body involvement, cell type, extravascular matrix patterns and cytogenetics

---

10.3.2 Retinoblastoma

Retinoblastoma is a malignant tumour of the immature retina. It is a rare malignancy with an incidence of 1 in 20,000 live births [107]. There is no gender or race predilection. The disease may occur in utero and up to the age of four years, the average age at appearance of first signs being seven months for bilateral cases and 24 months for unilateral cases [107]. Retinoblastoma occurs uncommonly in older children and exceptionally in young adults [107]. Although rare, retinoblastoma accounts for 80% of all primary ocular cancers in children up to 15 years old [107]. Fortunately, advances in therapy have improved survival to over 95% [107]. However, treatment at a late stage jeopardizes prognosis and hence emphasises the need for early diagnosis [107].

About two-thirds of all cases are unilateral and one-third of cases are bilateral [108]. Cases may be heritable or sporadic. Genetically, germline RB1 mutations have been identified in 91% of bilateral patients, 70% of familial unilateral patients and 7% of unilateral patients with no family history of the disease [109]. The "two-hit" hypothesis of oncogenesis with regards to somatic and germline mutations in retinoblastoma has been questioned recently, drawing attention to the role of epigenetic factors and aneuoploidy [110]. Patients with germline mutation retinoblastoma are at risk for neuroblastic intracranial malignancy in the first five years of life [108]. Patients with germline mutations are also at risk of second nonocular primary tumours occurring with a cumulative incidence of 1% per year [107].

10.3.2.1 Clinical Features

Leukocoria (60%) and strabismus (20%) are the most common presenting signs [107]. The remaining 20% of patients present atypical signs often masquerading as inflammation [107]. These atypical signs usually present late and are associated with a poorer prognosis [107]. Classically, early lesions appear as flat, transparent or slightly white, placoid masses within the neurosensory retina [98]. With enlargement, these tumours have a white appearance containing flecks of calcification [98].

Growth patterns may be endophytic towards the vitreous, exophytic spreading in the subretinal space, resulting in detachment, or a mixed growth pattern. In 2% of cases a diffuse infiltrating (plaque-like) growth pattern is observed with retinoblastoma developing in a flat irregular greyish plaque on or beneath the retina, progressing until the anterior segment is reached and pseudoinflammatory signs present, including pseudo-hypopyon [98, 107].

Other atypical presentations include spontaneous hyphaema, iris nodules or secondary glaucoma [98]. Tumour necrosis may produce anterior or posterior inflammation [98]. Tumour seeding into the vitreous cavity may be confused with an inflammatory vitritis [98]. Orbital inflammation may occur in the absence of orbital invasion mimicking an orbital cellulitis or panophthalmitis.

10.3.2.2 Diagnosis

The diagnosis of retinoblastoma can be made clinically by indirect ophthalmoscopy. If the fundus view is obscured, ultrasonography and computed tomography are indicated. Calcification is characteristic of retinoblastoma and is not frequently seen in other entities considered in the differential diagnosis. Diagnosis may be more difficult with inflammatory presentations, in particular diffuse infiltrative retinoblastoma. In this growth pattern, imaging investigations are less useful due to the absence of a tumour mass and a lower incidence of calcifications [98]. Intraocular diagnostic procedures are generally considered to be contraindicated due to the high risk of fatal iatrogenic seeding [98].

10.3.2.3 Management

Current first-line treatment approaches comprise systemic chemoreduction of lesions until they are amenable to adjuvant focal treatment methods. Focal treatment methods include cryotherapy, photocoagulation, chemothermotherapy, thermotherapy, brachytherapy, stereotactic conformal radiotherapy and accelerated proton beam irradiation [107]. Enucleation and external radiotherapy are now reserved for advanced cases [107]. The most significant risk factors for metastatic disease are optic nerve or orbital invasion and massive choroidal infiltration [107]. The International Classification of Retinoblastoma can reliably predict chemoreduction outcome based on tumour size, location and associated seeding. Excellent survival rates have been achieved with advances in treatment approaches.

Summary for the Clinician

- Treatment at a late stage jeopardizes prognosis and hence emphasises the need for early diagnosis
- 20% of patients present with atypical signs often masquerading as inflammation
- Intraocular diagnostic procedures are generally considered contraindicated due to the high risk of fatal iatrogenic seeding

---

10.3.3   Ocular Metastases

Metastatic tumours are the commonest intraocular malignancy in adults, but these rarely mimic intraocular inflammation. Most patients with metastatic ocular lesions are systemically ill with advanced disease and are not seen by the ophthalmologist. However, approximately one-third of patients have no history of primary cancer at the time of ocular diagnosis [111, 112]. Tumours metastasize to any ocular tissue. The uveal tract is most commonly affected, but retinal metastases are extremely rare [3]. Metastatic lesions may rarely be mistaken for intraocular inflammation [3].

Carcinomas are the most common primary lesions that produce ocular metastases [98]. The origin of primary tumour is gender dependent. Lung metastases are the most common in men and breast metastases are the most common in women [113]. In breast cancer, the primary tumour has been treated in 90% of cases by the time the ocular lesion presents [98]. In contrast, ocular metastases from renal and lung primaries may be the first presentation of disease in up to 80% of cases [98].

Ocular metastases are haematogenously disseminated. The choroid is the most frequent metastatic site on account of its rich vascular supply. It is affected approximately 10–20 times more often than the iris or ciliary body. The frequency of involvement of other ocular sites in patients with uveal metastases is described in Table 10.4 [112].

Table 10.4. Frequency of metastasis to other ocular sites in patients with uveal metastases ($n = 420$) [111]

Optic nerve	N = 24 (5%)
Conjunctiva	N = 8 (<1%)
Orbit	N = 7 (<1%)
Retina	N = 5 (<1%)
Eyelids	N = 3 (<1%)

10.3.3.1   Clinical Features

Iris and ciliary lesions are most likely to present diagnostic difficulty and masquerade [98]. Iris metastases arise most often from breast carcinoma, followed by carcinoma of the lung, carcinoid tumour and melanoma [113]. They present as unilateral lesions of varied colour, depending on the site of primary involvement [113]. The typical white or grey-white gelatinous nodule may be associated with iridocyclitis, secondary glaucoma, rubeosis, hyphaema or pupil irregularity [113]. Ciliary body tumours typically present as yellow sessile or dome-shaped masses [98]. They may induce iridocyclitis and spontaneous hyphaema [98]. Retinal metastases tend to be white with a perivascular distribution appearing similar to cotton-wool spots [113]. Progression of retinal lesions produces a singular well-circumscribed retinal mass [113]. The tumour cells seeding into the vitreous may mimic an inflammatory vitritis [113]. Lesions metastatic to the vitreous most commonly originate from cutaneous melanoma and lymphoproliferative disorders [113, 114]. They appear as clumps of pigmented or nonpigmented cells [113, 114]. Choroidal metastases are generally creamy yellow subretinal masses with overlying pigmentary changes that produce secondary retinal detachments [98].

10.3.3.2   Diagnosis

A careful medical history may be the key to diagnosis. Ocular metastases have been reported many years after primary removal, especially with carcinoid and renal tumours [98]. History and examination may suggest the correct diagnosis in most cases. However, if the primary tumour is unknown, the ophthalmic examination alone is unlikely to be diagnostic except in the rare case of a cutaneous melanoma metastatic to the eye in which brown pigment may be visible [98]. Of the patients with no known primary at the time of ocular presentation, the site of origin will never be identified in half [112]. Both fluorescein angiography and ultrasonography may help in delineating the borders of a choroidal tumour, but are of limited value in definitively differentiating these lesions from primary choroidal neoplasms [113]. Vitreous aspirates may be of use in making a diagnosis with ocular metastases of unknown primary [113]. The short-term prognosis for vision with ocular metastases is usually good, but the systemic prognosis is poor [111].

Summary for the Clinician

- Approximately one-third of patients have no history of primary cancer at the time of ocular diagnosis
- Metastatic lesions may rarely be mistaken for intraocular inflammation
- Ocular metastases have been reported many years after primary removal, especially with carcinoid and renal tumours

10.3.4 Juvenile Xanthogranuloma

Juvenile xanthogranuloma (JXG) is a rare histiocytic disorder. It is the commonest form of non-Langerhans' cell histiocytosis [115]. It is predominantly a disease of infancy, although adult onset is possible [116]. JXG is characterised by primarily cutaneous involvement, though other organs and tissues may also be affected [116]. The prognosis is generally benign, with cutaneous lesions undergoing spontaneous regression over several years [116]. However, CNS or other vital organ involvement and ocular involvement may be life- and sight-threatening [116]. The eye is the most frequently affected extracutaneous site. The incidence of eye involvement in patients with cutaneous JXG was estimated to be 0.3–0.5% [116]. In contrast, at least 41% of patients with ocular involvement had cutaneous lesions that were always multiple [116]. In up to 45% of patients with coexistent cutaneous JXG, skin lesions developed after those in the eye [116]. 51% of patients never develop skin lesions [117]. As a result, JXG may first present to the ophthalmologist [117].

10.3.4.1 Clinical Features

The eye is severely red and painful, mimicking inflammation. The characteristic skin lesions are firm rubbery papules or nodules with a reddish-yellow colour [3]. Ocular involvement occurs most often during the first 2 years of life but adult onset is also possible [116]. The most common ocular manifestations are a unilateral iris lesion, spontaneous hyphaema and potentially blinding secondary glaucoma [117]. The eyelid is the second most commonly affected site [116]. Patients may also present with an anterior uveitis or acquired heterochromia if iris involvement is diffuse [3]. Other ocular sites infrequently reported include conjunctiva, cornea, episclera, retina, choroid and optic nerve [117]. Posterior segment involvement may result in retinal detachment [3]. Rare cases of orbital involvement have been described [116].

10.3.4.2 Diagnosis

Ocular JXG requires prompt diagnosis and intervention in order to minimise complications [117]. Misdiagnosis can lead to inappropriate measures such as enucleation for presumed malignancy [117]. Tissue biopsy from skin lesions, aqueous tap, iris biopsy or excisional biopsy are useful for confirming clinical suspicions [117, 118].

Histologically, cutaneous lesions are classically described as a mass of large mononuclear cells with foamy cytoplasm with the presence of fat containing Touton-type giant cells [116]. The lipid contains apolipoprotein A and can be demonstrated with oil red O staining [116]. Iris lesion histiocytes show foamy cytoplasm and Touton giant cells less often than in skin lesions [117]. Newly formed thin-walled blood vessels are often present in the iris stroma [117]. Immunohistochemical findings may help diagnose atypical variants of JXG and differentiate JXG from other histiocytic disorders [116].

10.3.4.3 Management

Uveal lesions must be treated early due the risk of blinding secondary glaucoma [117]. Treatment of secondary glaucoma consists of aggressive topical and oral pressure-lowering agents [117]. Corneal or limbal lesions may be treated by local excision and or lamellar graft [118]. Intraocular and orbital lesions may respond to topical, peribulbar or systemic corticosteroid therapy [117]. Resistant cases may require irradiation or immunosuppression [3].

Summary for the Clinician

- The eye is the most frequently affected extracutaneous site
- JXG may first present to the ophthalmologist
- Ocular involvement occurs most often during the first two years of life
- The most common ocular manifestations are a unilateral iris lesion, spontaneous hyphaema and potentially blinding secondary glaucoma

References

1. Theodore FH (1967) Conjunctival carcinoma masquerading as chronic conjunctivitis. Eye Ear Nose Throat 46:1419–1420

2. Rothova A, Ooijman F, Kerkhoff F et al. (2001) Uveitis masquerade syndromes. Ophthalmology 108:386–399

3. Read RW, Zamir E, Raod NA (2002) Neoplastic masquerade syndromes. Surv Ophthalmol 47:81–124

4. Chan CC, Buggage RR, Nussenblatt RB (2002) Intraocular lymphoma. Curr Opin Ophthalmol 13:411–418

5. Chan CC, Wallace DJ (2004) Intraocular lymphoma: update on diagnosis and management. Cancer control 11:285–295

6. Choi JY, Kafkala C, Foster CS (2006) Primary intraocular lymphoma: a review. Semin Ophthalmol 21:125–133

7. Paulus W (1999) Classification, pathogenesis and molecular pathology of primary CNS lymphomas. J Neurooncol 43:203–208

8. Hoffman PM, McKelvie P, Hall AJ et al. (2003) Intraocular lymphoma: a series of 14 patients with clinicopathological features and treatment outcomes. Eye 17:513–521

9. Bardenstein DS (1998) Intraocular lymphoma. Cancer Control 5:317–325

10. Hochberg FH, Miller DC (1988) Primary central nervous system lymphoma. J Neurosurg 68:835–853

11. Schabet M (1999) Epidemiology of primary CNS lymphoma. J Neurooncol 43:199–201

12. Hochberg FH, Miller DC (1988) Primary central nervous system lymphoma. J Neurosurg 68:835–853

13. Nasir S, DeAngelis LM (2000) Update on the management of primary CNS lymphoma. Oncology 14:228–234

14. Wender A, Adar A, Maor E, Yassur Y (1994) Primary B-cell lymphoma of the eyes and brain in a 3-year old boy. Arch Ophthalmol 112:450–451

15. Freeman LN, Schachat AP, Knox DL et al. (1987) Clinical features, laboratory investigations, and survival in ocular reticulum cell sarcoma. Ophthalmology 94:1631–1639

16. Whitcup SM, de Smet MD, Rubin BL et al. (1993) Intraocular lymphoma. Clinical and histopathological diagnosis. Ophthalmology 100:1399–1406

17. Akpek EK, Ahmed L, Hochberg FH et al. (1999) Intraocular–central nervous system lymphoma: clinical features, diagnosis and outcomes. Ophthalmology 106:1805–1810

18. DeAngelis LM (2001) Brain tumours. New Engl J Med 344:114–123

19. Davis JL (2004) Diagnosis of intraocular lymphoma. Ocular Immunol Inflamm 12:7–16

20. Peterson K, Gordon KB, Heinemann MH et al. (1993) The clinical spectrum of ocular lymphoma. Cancer 72:843–849

21. Gill MK, Jampol LM (2001) Variations in the presentation of primary intraocular lymphoma: case reports and a review. Surv Ophthalmol 45:463–471

22. Velez G, Chan CC, Csaky KG (2002) Fluorescein angiographic findings in primary intraocular lymphoma. Retina 22:37–43

23. Graham E (1987) Intraocular involvement of T and B cell lymphomas. Eye 1:691–698

24. Velez G, de Smet MD, Whitcup SM et al. (2000) Iris involvement in primary intraocular lymphoma: report of two cases and review of the literature. Surv Ophthalmol 44:518–256

25. Lobo A, Larkin G, Clark BJ et al. (2003) Pseudo-hypopyon as the presenting feature in B-cell and T-cell intraocular lymphoma. Clin Exp Ophthalmol 31:155–158

26. Char DH, Ljung BM, Miller T et al. (1988) Primary intraocular lymphoma (ocular reticulum sarcoma) diagnosis and management. Ophthalmology 95:625–630

27. Buggage RR, Chan CC, Nussenblatt RB (2001) Ocular manifestations of central nervous system lymphoma. Curr Opin Oncol 13:137–142

28. de Smet MD, Nussenblatt RB, Davis JL, Palestine AG (1990) Large cell lymphoma masquerading as a viral retinitis. Int Ophthalmol 14:413–417

29. Ridley ME, McDonald HR, Sternberg P Jr et al. (1992) Retinal manifestations of ocular lymphoma (reticulum cell sarcoma). Ophthalmology 99:1153–1160

30. Levy-Clarke GA, Byrnes GA, Buggage RR et al. (2001) Primary intraocular lymphoma diagnosed by fine needle aspiration biopsy of a subretinal lesion. Retina 21:281–284

31. Gass JD, Trattler HL (1991) Retinal artery obstruction and atheromas associated with non-Hodgkins large cell lymphoma (reticulum cell sarcoma). Arch Ophthalmol 109:1134–1139

32. Brown SM, Jampol LM, Cantrill HL (1994) Intraocular lymphoma presenting as retinal vasculitis. Surv Ophthalmol 39:133–140

33. Balmaceda CM, Fetell MR, Selman JE, Seplowitz AJ (1994) Diabetes insipidus as first manifestation of primary central nervous system lymphoma. Neurology 44:358–359

34. Cassoux N, Merle-Beral H, Leblond V et al. (2000) Ocular and central nervous system lymphoma: clinical features and diagnosis. Ocular Immunol Inflamm 8:243–250

35. Ursea, Heinemann MH, Silverman RH et al. (1997) Ophthalmic, ultrasonographic findings in primary central nervous system lymphoma with ocular involvement. Retina 17:118–123

36. DeAngelis LM (1999) Primary central nervous system lymphoma. Curr Opin Neurol 12:687–691

37. Lobo A, Lightman S (2003) Vitreous aspiration needle tap in the diagnosis of intraocular inflammation. Ophthalmology 110:595–599

38. Merle-Beral H, Frederic D, Cassoux N et al. (2004) Biological diagnosis of primary intraocular lymphoma. Br J Haematol 124:469–473

39. Whitcup SM, Chan CC, Buggage RR et al. (2000) Improving the diagnostic yield of vitrectomy for intraocular lymphoma (Letter). Arch Ophthalmol 118:46

40. Pavan PR, Oteiza EE, Margo CE (1995) Ocular lymphoma diagnosed by internal subretinal pigment epithelium biopsy. Arch Ophthalmol 113:1233–1244

41. Kirmani MH, Thomas EL, Roa NA et al. (1987) Intraocular reticulum cell sarcoma: diagnosis by choroidal biopsy. Br J Ophthalmol 71:748–752

42. Zaldivar RA, Martin DF, Holden JT et al. (2004) Primary intraocular lymphoma: clinical, cytologic and flow cytometric analysis. Ophthalmology 111:1762–1767

43. Farkas T, Harbour JW, Davila RM (2004) Cytological diagnosis of intraocular lymphoma in vitreous aspirates. Acta Cytologica 48:487–491

44. Chan CC, Whitcup SM, Solomon D et al. (1995) Interleukin-10 in the vitreous of patients with primary intraocular lymphoma. Am J Ophthalmol 120:671–673

45. Davis JL, Solomon D, Nussenblatt RB et al. (1992) Immunocytochemical staining or vitreous cells. Indications, techniques and results. Ophthalmology 99:250–256

46. Coupland SE, Bechrakis NE, Anastassiou G et al. (2003) Evaluation of vitrectomy specimens and chorioretinal biopsies in the diagnosis of primary intraocular lymphoma in patients with masquerade syndrome. Graefe's Arch Clin Exp Ophthalmol 241:860–870

47. Wilson DJ, Braziel R, Rosenbaum JT (1992) Intraocular lymphoma. Immunopathologic analysis of vitreous biopsy specimens. Arch Ophthalmol 110:1455–1458

48. Whitcup SM, Stark-Vancs V, Wittes RE et al. (1997) Association of interleukin-10 in the vitreous and cerebrospinal fluid and primary central nervous system lymphoma. Arch Ophthalmol 115:1157–1160

49. Akpek EK, Maca SM, Christen WG et al. (1999) Elevated vitreous interleukin-10 is not diagnostic of intraocular–central nervous system lymphoma. Ophthalmology 106:2291–2295

50. Chan CC (2003) Molecular pathology of primary intraocular lymphoma. Trans Am Ophthalmol Soc 101:275–292

51. Shen DF, Zhuang A, LeHoang P et al. (1998) Utility of microdissection and polymerase chain reaction for the detection of immunoglobulin gene rearrangement and translocation in primary intraocular lymphoma. Ophthalmology 105:1664–1669

52. Katai N, Kuroiwa S, Fujimori K et al. (1997) Diagnosis of intraocular lymphoma by polymerase chain reaction. Graefes Arch Clin Exp Ophthlamol 235:431–436

53. Ferreri AJ, Blay JY, Reni M et al. (2002) Relevance of intraocular involvement in the management of primary central nervous system lymphomas [International Extranodal Lymphoma Study Group (IELSG)]. Ann Oncol 13:531–538

54. Abrey LE, DeAngelis LM, Yahalom J (1998) Long-term survival in primary CNS lymphoma. J Clin Oncol 16:859–863

55. Batchelor TT, Kolak G, Ciordia R et al. (2003) High-dose methotrexate for intraocular lymphoma. Clin Cancer Res 9:711–715

56. Mason JO, Fischer DH (2003) Intrathecal chemotherapy for recurrent central nervous system intraocular lymphoma. Ophthalmology 110:1241–1244

57. Sandor V, Stark-Vancs V, Pearson D et al. (1998) Phase II trial of chemotherapy alone for primary CNS and intraocular lymphoma. J Clin Oncol 16:3000–3006

58. de Smet MD (2001) Management of non Hodgkin's intraocular lymphoma with intravitreal methotrexate. Bullet de la Societe Belge d'Ophthalmologie 279:91–95

59. Soussain C, Suzan F, Hoang-Xuan K et al. (2001) Results of intensive chemotherapy followed by haematopoietic stem-cell rescue in 22 patients with refractory or recurrent primary CNS lymphoma or intraocular lymphoma. J Clin Oncol 19:742–749

60. Jahnke K, Bechrakis NE, Coupland SE et al. (2004) Treatment of primary intraocular lymphoma with oral trofosfamide: report of two cases and review of the literature. Graefes Arch Clin Exp Ophthalmol 242:771–776

61. Ben-Ezra D, Sahel JA, Harris NL et al. (1989) Uveal lymphoid infiltrates: immunohistochemical evidence for a lymphoid neoplasia. Br J Ophthalmol 73:846–851

62. Jakobiec FA, Sacks E, Kronish JW et al. (1987) Multifocal static creamy choroidal infiltrates. An early sign of lymphoid neoplasia. Ophthalmology 94:397–406

63. Harris NL, Jaffe ES, Stein H et al. (1994) A revised European-American classification of lymphoid neoplasms: a proposal from the International Lymphoma Study Group. Blood 84:1361–1392

64. Coupland SE, Foss HD, Hidayat AA et al. (2002) Extranodal marginal zone B cell lymphomas of the uvea: an analysis of 13 cases. J Pathol 197:333–340

65. Coupland SE, Joussen A, Anastassiou G et al. (2005) Diagnosis of a primary uveal extranodal marginal zone B-cell lymphoma by chorioretinal biopsy: case report. Graefe's Arch Clin Exp Ophthalmol 243:482–486

66. Cockeram GC, Hidayat AA, Bijwaard KE et al. (2000) Reevaulation of reactive lymphoid hyperplasia of the uvea: an immunohistochemical and molecular analysis of 10 cases. Ophthalmology 107:151–158

67. Coupland SE, Damato B (2006) Lymphomas involving the eye and the ocular adnexa. Curr Opin Ophthalmol 17:523–531

68. Parikh AH, Sameer HK, Wright JD et al. (2005) Systemic non-Hodgkin's lymphoma simulating primary intraocular lymphoma. Am J Ophthalmol 139:573–574

69. Barr CC, Joondeph HC (1983) Retinal periphlebitis as the initial clinical finding in a patient with Hodgkin's disease. Retina 3:253–257

10

70. Primbs GB, Monsees WE, Irvine AR (1961) Intraocular Hodgkin's disease. Arch Ophthalmol 66:477–482

71. Gunduz K, Shields JA, Shields CL (1999) Transscleral choroidal biopsy in the diagnosis of choroidal lymphoma. Surv Ophthalmol 43:551–555

72. Fredrick DR, Char DH, Ljung BM et al. (1989) Solitary intraocular lymphoma as an initial presentation of widespread disease. Arch Ophthalmol 107:395–397

73. Coupland SE, Loddenkemper C, Smith JR et al. (2005) Expression of immunoglobulin transcription factors in primary intraocular lymphoma and primary central nervous system lymphoma. Investig Ophthalmol Vis Sci 46:3957–3964

74. Mudhar H, Sethuraman C, Khan DM et al. (2007) Intraocular, pan-uveal intravascular large B-cell lymphoma choroidal infarction, and choroidal tri-lineage extramedullary haematopoiesis. Histopathology 51:275–279

75. Elner VM, Hidayat AA, Charles NC et al. (1986) Neoplastic angioentheliomatosis: a variant of malignant lymphoma: immunohistochemical and ultrastructural observations of three cases. Ophthalmology 93:1237–1245

76. Coupland SE, Anastassiou G, Bornfeld N et al. (2005) Primary intraocular lymphoma of T-cell type: report of a case and review of the literature. Graefe's Arch Clin Exp Ophthalmol 243:189–197

77. Goldey SH, Stern GA, Oblon DJ et al. (1989) Immunophenotypic characterization of an unusual T-cell lymphoma presenting as anterior uveitis. A clinicopathological case report. Arch Ophthalmol 107:1349–1353

78. Jensen OA, Johansen S, Kiss S (1994) Intraocular T-cell lymphoma mimicking a ring melanoma. First manifestation of a systemic disease. Report of a case and survery of the literature. Graefe's Arch Clin Exp Ophthalmol 232:148–152

79. Reim H, Dieler R, Wessing A (1990) Non-Hodgkin's lymphoma simulating chorioretinitis. Fortschritte der Ophthalmologie 87:557–559

80. Yeh KH, Lien HC, Hsu SM et al. (1999) Quiescent nasal T/NK cell lymphoma manifested as primary central nervous system lymphoma. Am J Haematol 60:161–163

81. Hon C, Kwok AK, Shek TW et al. (2002) Vision-threatening complications of nasal T/NK lymphoma. Am J Ophthalmol 134:406–410

82. Leitch RJ, Rennie IG, Parsons MA (1993) Ocular involvement in mycosis fungoides. Br J Ophthalmol 77:126–127

83. Keltner JL, Fritsch E, Cykiert RC et al. (1977) Mycosis fungoides: intraocular and central nervous system involvement. Arch Ophthalmol 95:645–650

84. Erny BC, Egbert PR, Peat IM et al. (1991) Intraocular involvement with subretinal pigment epithelial infiltrates by mycosis fungoides. Br J Ophthalmol 75:698–701

85. Lois N, Hiscott PS, Nash J et al. (2000) Immunophenotypic shift in a case of mycosis fungoides with vitreous invasion. Arch Ophthalmol 118:1692–1694

86. Woog J, Kim YD, Yeatts RP et al. (2006) Natural killer/T-cell lymphoma with ocular and adnexal involvement. Ophthalmology 113:140–147

87. Coupland SE, Foss HD, Assaf C et al. (1999) T-cell and T/natural killer cell lymphomas involving ocular and ocular adnexal tissues. Ophthalmology 106:2109–2120

88. Kohno T, Uchida H, Inomata H et al. (1993) Ocular manifestations of adult T-cell leukaemia/lymphoma. Ophthalmology 100:1794–1799

89. Kumar SR, Gill PS, Wagner DG et al. (1994) Human T-cell lymphotrophic virus type I-associated retinal lymphoma. A clinicopathologic report. Arch Ophthalmol 112:954–959

90. Davis JL, Miller DM, Ruiz P (2005) Diagnostic testing of vitrectomy specimens. Am J Ophthalmol 140:829–899

91. Kincaid MC, Green R (1983) Ocular and orbital involvement in leukaemia. Surv Ophthalmol 27:211–232

92. Hattenhauer MG, Pach JM (1996) Ocular lymphoma in a patient with chronic lymphocytic leukaemia. Am J Ophthalmol 122:266–268

93. Coupland SE, Foss HD, Bechrakis NE et al. (2001) Secondary ocular involvement in systemic "memory" B-cell lymphocytic leukaemia. Ophthalmology 108:1289–1295

94. Tranos PG, Andreou PS, Wickremasinghe SS et al. (2002) Pseudohypopyon as a feature of multiple myeloma. Arch Ophthalmol 120:87–88

95. Knapp AJ, Gartner S, Henkind P (1987) Multiple myeloma and its ocular manifestations. Surv Ophthalmol 31:343–351

96. Shakin EP, Augsburger JJ, Eagle RC et al. (1988) Multiple melanoma involving the iris. Arch Ophthalmol 106:524–526

97. Singh AD, Bergman L, Seregard S (2005) Uveal melanoma: epidemiological aspects. Ophthalmol Clin N Am 18:75–84

98. Tsai T, O'Brien JM (2002) Masquerade syndromes: malignancies mimicking inflammation in the eye. Int Ophthalmol Clin 42:115–131

99. Damato B (2004) Developments in the management of uveal melanoma. Clin Exp Ophthalmol 32:639–647

100. Simpson ER (2004) Ciliary body melanoma: a special challenge. Can J Ophthalmol 39:365–371

101. Wanner JB, Pasquale LR (2006) Glaucomas secondary to intraocular melanomas. Semin Ophthlamol 21:181–189

102. Collaborative Ocular Melanoma Study Group (1990) Accuracy of diagnosis of choroidal melanomas in the Collaborative Ocular Melanoma Study (COMS report no. 1). Arch Ophthalmol 108:1268–1273

103. Bakri SJ, Sculley L, Singh AD (2006) Imaging techniques for uveal melanoma. Int Ophthalmol Clin 46:1–13

104. Shields JA (2002) Management of posterior uveal melanoma: past, present and future. Retina 22:139–142

105. Baggetto LG, Gambrelle J, Dayan G (2005) Major cytogenetic aberrations and typical multidrug resistance phenotype of uveal melanoma: current views and new therapeutic prospects. Cancer Treatment Rev 31:361–379

106. Kujala E, Makitie T, Kivela T (2003) Very long term prognosis of patients with malignant uveal melanoma. Investig Ophthalmol Vis Sci 44:4651–4659

107. Balmer A, Zografos L, Munier F (2006) Diagnosis and current management of retinoblastoma. Oncogene 25:5341–5349

108. Shields CL, Shields JA (2006) Basic understanding of current classification and management of retinoblastoma. Curr Opin Ophthalmol 17:228–234

109. Nichols KE, Houseknecht MD, Godmilow L et al. (2005) Sensitive multistep clinical molecular screening of 180 unrelated individuals with retinoblastoma detects 36 novel mutations in the RB1 gene. Hum Mutations 25:566–574

110. Mastrangelo D, Francesco SD, Leonardo AD et al. (2007) Retinoblastoma epidemiology: does the evidence matter? Eur J Cancer 43:1596–1603

111. Potter PD (1998) Ocular manifestations of cancer. Curr Opin Ophthalmol 9:100–104

112. Shields CL, Shields JA, Gross NE et al. (1997) Survey of 520 eyes with uveal metastases. Ophthalmology 104:1265–1276

113. Solomon S, Smith JH, O'Brien J (1999) Ocular manifestations of systemic malignancies. Curr Opin Ophthalmol 10:447–451

114. Gunduz K, Shields JA, Shields CL et al. (1998) Cutaneous melanoma metastatic to the vitreous. Ophthalmology 105:600–605

115. Weitzman S, Jaffe R (2005) Uncommon histiocytic disorders: the non-Langerhans cell histiocytoses. Pediatr Blood Cancer 45:256–264

116. Hernandez-Martin A, Baselga E, Drolet BA et al. (1997) Juvenile xanthogranuloma. J Am Acad Dermatol 36:355–367

117. Vendal Z, Walton D, Chen T (2006) Glaucoma in juvenile xanthogranuloma. Semin Ophthalmol 21:191–194

118. Chaudhry IA, Al-Jishi Z, Shamsi F et al. (2004) Juvenile xanthogranuloma of the corneoscleral limbus: case report and review of the literature. Surv Ophthalmol 49:608–614

Index

Printing and Binding: Stürtz GmbH, Würzburg